Also by Corinne T. Netzer:

THE DIETER'S CALORIE COUNTER
THE BRAND-NAME CALORIE COUNTER
THE COMPLETE BOOK OF FOOD COUNTS
THE FAT CONTENT OF FOOD
THE CORINNE T. NETZER ENCYCLOPEDIA OF FOOD VALUES
THE CORINNE T. NETZER DIETER'S DIARY
THE BRAND-NAME CARBOHYDRATE GRAM COUNTER
THE CORINNE T. NETZER 1992 CALORIE COUNTER

THE
CHOLESTEROL
CONTENT
OF
FOOD

(Revised Edition)
Corinne T. Netzer

A DELL BOOK

Published by
Dell Publishing
a division of
Bantam Doubleday Dell Publishing Group, Inc.
666 Fifth Avenue
New York, New York 10103

For my friends
at The Pierre
C.N.

ISBN: 0-440-20739-8

Printed in the United States of America

Published simultaneously in Canada

April 1992

10 9 8 7 6 5 4 3 2 1

OPM

Introduction

WHAT IS CHOLESTEROL?

Cholesterol, an essential fatlike substance present in all animal life, is found among fats in the bloodstream. When cholesterol builds up in the lining of the blood vessels over a period of time, these blood vessels can narrow or close. If the arteries supplying blood to the heart, brain, or other crucial organs are blocked, the result can be heart attack, stroke, or failure of other vital organs.

The body gets cholesterol from two sources. Each day the liver manufactures about 1,000 milligrams of cholesterol, which is needed to produce certain hormones and to construct cells. The remaining cholesterol in the body comes from dietary sources. Because the body manufactures all it needs, it is the added dietary cholesterol that concerns us.

WHO SHOULD REDUCE CHOLESTEROL?

After an eighteen-month study, a federal health panel of twenty-two expert members concluded that large amounts of cholesterol can lead to heart disease, and that there should be an aggressive attack on high blood cholesterol to reduce the national risk. The panel warned that forty million Americans have high cholesterol levels, placing them at high risk of heart disease.

The National Heart, Lung and Blood Institute report states that about twenty-five percent of Americans between the ages of twenty and seventy-four have high blood cholesterol and need treatment.

According to the National Institutes of Health, approximately 1.5 million Americans suffer heart attacks each year, and 500,000 die.

GUIDELINES TO REDUCING CHOLESTEROL

The federal panel stated that the desirable blood cholesterol level is 200 milligrams per deciliter, or less. The recommendation is that people with these readings have their cholesterol level rechecked every five years.

People with readings from 200 to 239 milligrams should be treated if they have other risk factors, the experts said. That recommendation includes every man with a reading over 200, because being male is one risk factor. Other risk factors include smoking, family history of heart disease, the presence of high blood pressure or diabetes, a history of stroke or blockage of blood vessels, and severe obesity.

Everyone with a reading of 240 milligrams or higher should be treated.

The recommendations were based on studies showing that every 1 percent reduction in blood cholesterol readings is accompanied by a 2 percent reduction in heart attack deaths.

THE RECOMMENDED DIET

The federal-recommended diet for reducing cholesterol starts with the *STEP 1 DIET,* which consists of reducing total fat in the diet to less than thirty percent of calorie intake, saturated fat to less than ten percent of calories, and cholesterol to less than 300 milligrams per day. This diet is generally consistent with previous recommendations of the American Heart Association.

If the *STEP 1 DIET* fails to achieve the desired goals, the person is to be put on a *STEP 2 DIET* that reduces saturated fat to less than seven percent of total calories and cholesterol intake to less than 200 milligrams per day.

If six months of dieting does not do the job, drugs are to be considered in addition to the diet. These drugs are unpleasant and may have severe side effects, so strict adherence to the diet is the best course.

HOW THIS BOOK CAN HELP YOU LOWER CHOLESTEROL

The Cholesterol Content of Food is designed to take the guesswork out of cholesterol dieting.

Plan what you are going to have for the day, or even for the week. Then just look up the cholesterol content—listings are arranged alphabetically for instant reference—and add up the figures. If you have chosen a 300-milligrams-of-cholesterol-per-day diet and you're over 300 milligrams a day, you have to make an adjustment and decrease your cholesterol intake. If you choose the 200-milligram-a-day diet, you must make a similar adjustment. It's that simple; and yet that hard, because at first you may find it troublesome. After all, many of the things we love most are high in cholesterol. But the benefits far outweigh the dietary inconvenience.

Lowering your cholesterol intake may lower your blood cholesterol count, but you should try to think of this as a new and better way of life, not just a stopgap temporary measure. I have, and I'm very proud of myself. You will be too.

CHOLESTEROL AND DIETARY FAT

Just because you look up a listing for a fat and it indicates that there is no cholesterol content does not mean that this is good for your diet. It is important for you to know that you should limit your intake of saturated fats because *they can raise your blood cholesterol level.*

Curtail your intake of coconut and palm oils; they are highly saturated. Also cut down on foods containing hydrogenated oils, since hydrogenation makes fats more saturated.

You may see a product on your supermarket shelf that claims to be cholesterol-free because it uses only vegetable oil. Don't assume that cholesterol-free means heart healthy. Read labels. For instance, I'm sure you've read this listing on a box: "Contains one or more of the following: soybean, hydrogenated cottonseed, and/or palm kernel oil." This gives the manufacturer a choice when prices fluctuate. When presented with such a list assume the worst, since saturated oils tend to be cheaper and have a longer shelf life.

THE DATA IN THIS BOOK

Unless otherwise indicated, listings for cooked generic foods are baked, boiled, broiled, etc. *without added ingredients,* and brand-name foods that require preparation are *prepared according to basic package directions.*

All information in this book is based on data supplied by the United States government or the individual producers and manufacturers.

As we go to press, *The Cholesterol Content of Food* contains the most complete and up-to-date listings of cholesterol in food. In the future, as more information becomes available, I will be updating and revising this book.

Good luck and good dieting.

Corinne T. Netzer

Abbreviations

diam.	diameter
fl.	fluid
lb.	pound
mgs.	milligrams
oz.	ounce
pkg.	package
pkt.	packet
tbsp.	tablespoon
tsp.	teaspoon
tr.	trace
w/	with
"	inch
<	less than
*	prepared according to package directions

A

Food and Measure	Cholesterol (mgs.)
Abalone, meat only:	
raw, 1 oz.	24
floured, fried in vegetable oil, 4 oz.	107
Acapulco dip:	
(Ortega)	0
Acerola:	
fresh	0
Acerola juice:	
fresh	0

Acorn squash:
raw, cooked, or frozen, w/out sauce   0

Adzuki beans:
cooked or canned   0

Albacore, see "Tuna, canned"

Alfalfa sprouts:
raw or cooked   0

Alfredo sauce:
canned *(Progresso* Authentic Pasta Sauces),
$^1/_2$ cup   95
refrigerated *(Contadina Fresh),* 6 oz.   85

Allspice:
berries or ground   0

Almond:
all varieties, raw, dried, or roasted   0

Almond butter or paste:
all varieties   0

Almond meal:
partially defatted   0

Amaranth:
raw or cooked   0

Anise seed:
whole or ground   0

Apple:
all varieties, fresh, canned, or dried   0

Apple, glazed, frozen:
   in raspberry sauce *(The Budget Gourmet),* 5 oz. . . . 10

Apple butter:
   all varieties 0

Apple cider, drink, or juice:
   all blends (all brands) 0

Apple cobbler:
   deep dish *(Awrey's)* 0

Apple crisp, frozen:
   (Pepperidge Farm Berkshire), 1 cup 40

Apple danish:
   (Awrey's Round), 2.75 oz. 5
   frozen *(Sara Lee Free & Light),* 1/8 pkg. 0
   frozen, twist *(Sara Lee),* 1/8 pkg. 10

Apple fritter, frozen:
   (Mrs. Paul's), 2 pieces 5

Apple pie spice:
   (Tone's) 0

Apple roll or snack, see "Fruit snack"

Apple sticks, frozen:
   (Farm Rich) 0

Applesauce:
   all varieties and blends (all brands) 0

Apricot:
   fresh, canned, dried, or frozen 0

Apricot nectar:
  (all brands) 0

Arby's, 1 serving:
  sandwiches:
    beef 'n cheddar 63
    chicken breast 91
    ham 'n cheese 45
    roast beef, regular 39
    roast beef, super 40
    roast chicken club 80
    turkey deluxe 39
  potato cakes, 3 oz. 0
  french fries, 2.5 oz. 0
  shake, Jamocha 35

Arrowhead:
  raw or cooked 0

Arrowroot flour:
  1 cup 0

Arthur Treacher's, 1 serving:
  chicken, 2 patties 65
  chicken sandwich 32
  chips, 4 oz. . . . . <85
  coleslaw 7
  fish, 2 pieces 56
  fish sandwich 42
  Krunch Pup 25
  Lemon Luvs . . . . <1
  shrimp, 7 pieces 93

Artichoke, globe:
  fresh, canned, or frozen, w/out sauce 0

Artichoke, Jerusalem, see "Jerusalem artichoke"

The Cholesterol Content of Food

Asparagus:
  fresh, canned, or frozen, w/out sauce   0

Asparagus pilaf, frozen:
  (Green Giant Microwave Garden Gourmet), 1 pkg.   10

Au jus gravy:
  canned *(Franco-American)*   0
  mix* *(French's)*   0

Avocado:
  California or Florida   0

Avocado dip:
  (Kraft)   0

B

Food and Measure	Cholesterol (mgs.)
Bacon, cooked:	
4.5 oz. (1 lb. raw)	107
(JM), 2 slices	12
(Oscar Mayer), 1 slice	5
(Oscar Mayer Center Cut/Lower Salt)*, 1 slice	6
(Oscar Mayer Thick Sliced)*, 1 slice	9
Bacon, Canadian:	
1 oz., unheated	14
(Jones Dairy Farm), 1 unheated slice	7
(Oscar Mayer), .8-oz. slice	11
Bacon, substitute:	
beef *(JM)*, 2 slices	20
turkey *(Louis Rich)*, 1 heated slice	10

The Cholesterol Content of Food

"Bacon," vegetarian, frozen:
(*Morningstar Farms* Breakfast Strips) 0
(*Worthington Stripples*) 0

Bacon bits:
(*Oscar Mayer*), 1/4 oz. 6
imitation (*Bac*Os*), 2 tsp. 0

Bacon and horseradish dip:
(*Breakstone's/Sealtest*), 2 tbsp. 15
(*Kraft*), 2 tbsp. 0
(*Kraft* Premium), 2 tbsp. 15

Bacon and onion dip:
(*Breakstone's* Gourmet), 2 tbsp. 15
(*Kraft* Premium), 2 tbsp. 15

Bagel, frozen, 1 piece:
all varieties, except egg and soft (*Lender's/
Lender's* Bagelettes/Big'n Crusty) 0
all varieties, except egg (*Sara Lee*) 0
egg:
(*Lender's*), 2 oz. 5
(*Lender's* Big'n Crusty), 31/8 oz. 15
(*Sara Lee*), 3.1 oz. 20
(*Sara Lee*), 2.5 oz. 15
soft (*Lender's*), 2.5 oz. 12

Baked beans, canned, 8 oz., except as noted:
(*Grandma Brown's*), 1 cup . . . . <1
(*Grandma Brown's* Saucepan), 1 cup . . . . <1
barbecue (*B&M*) 5
w/franks (*Van Camp's Beanee Weenee*), 1 cup . . . 15
honey (*B&M*) 0
hot and spicy (*B&M*) 3
maple (*B&M/Friends*) . . . . <5
pea beans (*B&M*) 5
pea beans, small (*Friends*) 6
w/pork (*Hormel Micro-Cup*), 7.5 oz. 30
red kidney (*Friends*) 4

Baked beans *(cont.)*
red kidney or small red *(B&M)* 5
tomato *(B&M)*. 1
vegetarian *(B&M)* 0
yellow eye *(B&M)* 4

Baking powder or soda:
(all brands) 0

Balsam-pear:
leafy-tips or pods, raw or boiled 0

Bamboo shoots:
fresh or canned (all brands) 0

Banana:
all varieties, fresh or dehydrated 0
chips, freeze-dried *(Mountain House)* 0

Banana nectar:
(Libby's) 0

Barbecue loaf:
(Oscar Mayer), 1-oz. slice 14

Barbecue sauce, 1 tbsp.:
(Hunt Original) 0
(Ott's) . . . . <1
all varieties *(Heinz/Heinz Thick and Rich)* 0
all varieties *(Kraft/Kraft Thick'N Spicy)* 0
all varieties *(Maull's)* . . . . <1
Cajun *(Golden Dipt)* 0
honey *(Hain)* 0
Oriental *(La Choy)* 0
original or mesquite *(Enrico's)* 0

Barley:
regular or pearled (all brands) 0

The Cholesterol Content of Food

Basil:
  fresh or dried 0

Baskin-Robbins:
  ice, daiquiri, 1 regular scoop 0
  ice cream, 1 regular scoop:
    almond fudge 32
    chocolate 37
    chocolate, *World Class* 36
    chocolate chip 40
    chocolate raspberry truffle, *International Cream* 45
    pralines 'n cream 36
    rocky road 32
    strawberry 30
    vanilla 52
    vanilla, French 90
  sherbet, rainbow, 1 regular scoop 6
  sorbet, red raspberry, 1 regular scoop 0
  cone, sugar or waffle, 1 piece 0

Bass, meat only (see also "Sea bass"):
  freshwater, raw, 1 lb. 308
  freshwater, raw, 1 oz. 19
  striped, raw, 1 lb. 363
  striped, raw, 1 oz. 20

Batter mix (see also specific listings):
  (Golden Dipt/Golden Dipt Corny Dog) 0

Bay leaf:
  dried (all brands) 0

Bean dip:
  hot or Mexican *(Hain)*, 4 tbsp. 5

Bean salad, canned:
  three bean *(Green Giant)* 0

Bean sprouts:
  all varieties, fresh or canned 0

Beans, see specific bean listings

Beans, snap or string, see "Green beans"

Beans, refried, see "Refried beans"

Beans and frankfurter dinner, frozen:
(Banquet), 10 oz.	35
(Morton), 10 oz.	30

Béarnaise sauce mix:
dry, .9-oz. pkt.	tr.

Beechnut:
dried	0

Beef,[1] choice, meat only, 4 oz., except as noted.:
brisket, whole, lean w/fat, braised	107
brisket, whole, lean only, braised	105
chuck:	
arm pot roast, lean w/fat, braised	112
arm pot roast, lean only, braised	115
blade roast, lean w/fat, braised	117
blade roast, lean only, braised	120
flank steak, 0" trim, lean only, braised	82
ground, raw:	
extra lean, 1 oz.	19
lean, 1 oz.	21
regular, 1 oz.	24
ground, broiled, medium:	
extra lean	95
lean	99
regular	102
porterhouse steak, lean w/fat, broiled	94
porterhouse steak, lean only, broiled	91

[1] *Retail trim to 1/4" fat, except as noted; cooked beef prepared without added ingredients.*

The Cholesterol Content of Food

rib:

    whole (ribs 6–12), lean w/fat, roasted 96
    whole (ribs 6–12), lean only, roasted 91
    large end (ribs 6–9), lean w/fat, roasted 96
    large end (ribs 6–9), lean only, roasted 92
    small end (ribs 10–12), lean w/fat, broiled 95
    small end (ribs 10–12), lean only, broiled 90

round:

    bottom, lean w/fat, braised 109
    bottom, lean only, braised 109
    eye of, lean w/fat, roasted 82
    eye of, lean only, roasted 78
    full cut, lean w/fat, broiled 91
    full cut, lean only, broiled 88
    tip, lean w/fat, roasted 94
    tip, lean only, roasted 92
    top, lean w/fat, broiled 96
    top, lean only, broiled 95
    top, lean w/fat, fried 110
    top, lean only, fried 110

shank, crosscuts, lean w/fat, simmered 91
shank, crosscuts, lean only, simmered 88
short ribs, lean w/fat, braised 107
short ribs, lean only, braised 105

sirloin, top:

    lean w/fat, broiled 102
    lean only, broiled 101
    lean w/fat, fried 111
    lean only, fried 112

T-bone steak, lean w/fat, broiled 94
T-bone steak, lean only, broiled 91
tenderloin, lean w/fat, broiled 98
tenderloin, lean only, broiled 95
top loin, lean w/fat, broiled 90
top loin, lean only, broiled 86

Beef, corned:

    (Healthy Deli), 1 oz. 11

Beef, corned *(cont.)*
  (Healthy Deli St. Paddy's), 1 oz. 7
  (Oscar Mayer), .6-oz. slice 8
  brisket, cured, cooked, 4 oz. 111

Beef, roast, see "Beef" and "Beef luncheon meat"

Beef, roast, spread:
  (Underwood Light), 2 1/8 oz. 30
  regular or mesquite smoke *(Underwood)*, 2 1/8 oz. 45

"Beef," vegetarian:
  canned or frozen, all varieties *(Worthington)* 0

Beef dinner, frozen:
  (Banquet Extra Helping), 16 oz. 120
  chopped *(Banquet)*, 11 oz. 80
  enchilada, see "Enchilada dinner"
  meat loaf, see "Meat loaf dinner"
  Mexicana *(The Budget Gourmet)*, 12.8 oz. 50
  patty, cheese, sandwich *(Kid Cuisine)*, 6.25 oz. . . . 40
  pepper steak *(Armour Classics Lite)*, 11.25 oz. . . . 35
  pepper steak *(Healthy Choice)*, 11 oz. 65
  pot roast, Yankee:
    (Armour Classics), 10 oz. 85
    (The Budget Gourmet), 11 oz. 70
    (Healthy Choice), 11 oz. 45
  Salisbury steak:
    (Armour Classics), 11.25 oz. 55
    (Armour Classics Lite), 11.5 oz. 35
    (Banquet), 11 oz. 80
    (Banquet Extra Helping), 18 oz. 175
    (Healthy Choice), 11.5 oz. 50
    (Le Menu LightStyle), 10 oz. 35
    (Morton), 10 oz. 40
    w/mushroom gravy *(Banquet Extra Helping)*,
      18 oz. 169
    parmigiana *(Armour Classics)*, 11.5 oz. 60

sirloin *(The Budget Gourmet)*, 11.5 oz. 105
short ribs *(Armour Classics)*, 9.75 oz. 90
sirloin:
  roast *(Armour Classics)*, 10.45 oz. 55
  tips *(Armour Classics)*, 10.25 oz. 70
  tips *(Healthy Choice)*, 11.75 oz. 70
  tips, in Burgundy sauce *(The Budget Gourmet)*,
    11 oz. 65
sliced *(Morton)*, 10 oz. 65
steak Diane *(Armour Classics Lite)*, 10 oz. 80
Stroganoff *(Armour Classics Lite)*, 11.25 oz. 55
Swiss steak *(The Budget Gourmet)*, 11.2 oz. 70

Beef entrée, canned or packaged:
chow mein *(La Choy Bi-Pack)*, 3/4 cup 20
pepper Oriental *(La Choy Bi-Pack)*, 3/4 cup 18
pepper steak, Oriental *(Hormel Top Shelf)*,
  1 serving 45
ribs, boneless *(Hormel Top Shelf)*, 1 serving 90
roast, tender *(Hormel Top Shelf)*, 1 serving 65
Salisbury steak, w/potatoes *(Hormel Top Shelf)*,
  10 oz. 88
stew *(Hormel/Dinty Moore Micro-Cup)*, 7.5 oz. . . . 50
Stroganoff *(Hormel Top Shelf)*, 1 serving 48
sukiyaki *(Hormel Top Shelf)*, 1 serving 45

Beef entrée, frozen:
(Banquet Platter), 10 oz. 75
and broccoli, w/rice *(La Choy Fresh & Lite)*, 11 oz. 51
cheeseburger *(MicroMagic)*, 4.75 oz. 80
Dijon, w/pasta and vegetables *(Right Course)*,
  9.5 oz. 40
enchilada, see "Enchilada entree"
fiesta, w/corn pasta *(Right Course)*, 8 7/8 oz. 30
hamburger *(MicroMagic)*, 4 oz. 55
London broil, in mushroom sauce *(Weight
  Watchers)*, 7.37 oz. 40
Oriental *(The Budget Gourmet Slim Selects)*, 10 oz. 25

Beef entrée, frozen *(cont.)*
  Oriental, w/vegetables and rice *(Lean Cuisine)*,
    8⅝ oz. 45
  pepper steak:
    (Dining Lite), 9 oz. 40
    (Healthy Choice), 9.5 oz. 40
    w/rice *(The Budget Gourmet)*, 10 oz. 25
    w/rice and vegetables *(La Choy Fresh & Lite)*,
      10 oz. 36
  pie:
    (Banquet), 7 oz. 25
    (Banquet Supreme Microwave), 7 oz. 35
    (Morton), 7 oz. 30
  pot roast *(Right Course)*, 9.25 oz. 35
  ragout, w/rice pilaf *(Right Course)*, 10 oz. 50
  Salisbury steak:
    (Dining Lite), 9 oz. 55
    w/Italian style sauce and vegetables *(Lean
      Cuisine)*, 9.5 oz. 100
    Romana *(Weight Watchers)*, 8.75 oz. 40
    sirloin *(The Budget Gourmet* Slim Selects), 9 oz. 75
  sirloin:
    in herb sauce *(The Budget Gourmet* Slim
      Selects), 10 oz. 25
    roast *(The Budget Gourmet)*, 9.5 oz. 85
    tips, w/country style vegetables *(The Budget
      Gourmet)*, 10 oz. 40
    tips and mushrooms, in wine sauce *(Weight
      Watchers)*, 7.5 oz. 50
  steak ranchero *(Lean Cuisine)*, 9.25 oz. 40
  Stroganoff *(The Budget Gourmet* Slim Selects),
    8.75 oz. 60
  Stroganoff *(Weight Watchers)*, 9 oz. 25
  Szechuan, w/noodles and vegetables *(Lean
    Cuisine)*, 9.25 oz. 100
  teriyaki *(Dining Lite)*, 9 oz. 45
  teriyaki, w/rice and vegetables *(La Choy Fresh &
    Lite)*, 10 oz. 57

Beef gravy, canned:
1/4 cup   2

Beef jerky:
(Frito-Lay's), .21 oz.   10
(Frito-Lay's Tender), .7 oz.   25

Beef luncheon meat:
roast:
    (Healthy Deli), 1 oz.   13
    (Oscar Mayer Thin Sliced), .4-oz. slice   5
    Italian *(Healthy Deli)*, 1 oz.   16
    top round *(Boar's Head)*, 1 oz.   20
    top round *(Boar's Head* Deluxe), 1 oz.   20
smoked *(Oscar Mayer)*, .5-oz. slice   7

Beef marinade seasoning mix:
(Lawry's)   0

Beef pie, see "Beef entree, frozen"

Beef roll or stick, see "Beef jerky"

Beef stew, see "Beef entree, canned or packaged"

Beef stew seasoning mix:
(French's)   0
(Lawry's)   0

Beefalo, meat only:
roasted, 4 oz.   66

Beer, ale, and malt liquor:
all varieties (all brands)   0

Beer batter mix:
(Golden Dipt), 1 oz.   0

Beet:
  plain or pickled, fresh or canned 0

Beet greens:
  raw or cooked 0

Berliner:
  pork and beef, 1 oz. 13

Berry drink or juice:
  all varieties (all brands) 0

Biscuit, 1 piece, except as noted:
  all varieties *(Awrey's)* 0
  frozen *(Bridgford),* 2 oz. 1
  mix* *(Martha White BixMix)* 1
  refrigerated, all varieties:
    (Ballard Ovenready) 0
    (Big Country/Big Country Butter Tastin') 0
    (1869 Brand) 0
    (Hungry Jack) 0
    (Pillsbury) 0

Black beans:
  cooked or canned (all brands) 0

Blackberry:
  fresh, canned, or frozen 0

Black-eyed peas, see "Cowpeas"

Blood sausage:
  1 oz. 34

Bloody Mary cocktail mix:
  bottled *(Holland House* Smooth N' Spicy) 0

Blue cheese dip, see "Cheese dip"

Blueberry:
fresh, canned, or frozen 0

Blueberry cobbler:
deep dish *(Awrey's)* 0

Bluefish, meat only:
raw, 1 lb. 266
raw, 1 oz. 17

Bok choy, see "Cabbage"

Bologna, 1 oz., except as noted:
(Boar's Head) 15
(Boar's Head Lower Salt) 20
(Eckrich Lite) 15
(Oscar Mayer), .53-oz. slice 10
(Oscar Mayer) 19
(Oscar Mayer), 1.6-oz. slice 31
(Oscar Mayer Light) 11
(Oscar Mayer Light), 1.4-oz. slice 16
w/cheese *(Oscar Mayer)*, .8-oz. slice 15
beef:
  (Boar's Head) 17
  (Hebrew National Original Deli Style) 15
  (Oscar Mayer), .53-oz. slice 10
  (Oscar Mayer) 19
  (Oscar Mayer), 1.6-oz. slice 31
  (Oscar Mayer Light) 10
  garlic flavor *(Oscar Mayer)* 18
  garlic flavor *(Oscar Mayer)*, 1.4-oz. slice 26
  Lebanon *(Oscar Mayer)*, .8-oz. slice 16
beef and pork *(Healthy Deli)* 9
turkey, see "Turkey bologna"

"Bologna," vegetarian, frozen:
(Worthington Bolono) 0

Bolognese sauce:
canned *(Progresso* Authentic Pasta Sauces),
1/2 cup 20
refrigerated *(Contadina Fresh),* 7.5 oz. 50

Borage:
raw or cooked 0

Bouillon (see also "Soup"):
onion or vegetable, instant *(Wyler's)* 0

Boysenberry:
fresh, canned, or frozen 0

Boysenberry juice:
(Smucker's Naturally 100%) 0

Brains:
beef, fried, 4 oz. 2262
lamb, fried, 4 oz. 2840
pork, braised, 4 oz. 2894
veal, fried, 4 oz. 2404

Bran, see "Oat bran" and "Wheat bran"

Bratwurst:
pork, cooked, 1 oz. 17
smoked *(Eckrich Lite* Bratwurst Links), 1 link 60

Braunschweiger:
(Oscar Mayer German Brand), 1 oz. 45
(Oscar Mayer Slices), 1 oz. 50
(Oscar Mayer Slices), .9-oz. slice 47
(Oscar Mayer Tube), 1 oz. 47

Brazil nut:
dried 0

The Cholesterol Content of Food

Bread, 1 slice:

 all varieties:
   (Monk's) 0
   (Oatmeal Goodness) 0
   (Pepperidge Farm) 0
   (Roman Light/Roman Meal) 0
   (Wonder) 0
 apple walnut *(Arnold)* 1
 (Arnold/Brownberry Bran'nola) . . . . tr.
 bran, whole *(Brownberry* Natural) 0
 cinnamon raisin *(Arnold)* 2
 corn, see "Cornbread mix"
 French, extra sour, sliced *(Colombo* Brand) 0
 grain, nutty *(Arnold/Brownberry Bran'nola)* . . . . . . tr.
 Italian:
   (Brownberry Light) . . . . tr.
   all varieties *(Arnold* Francisco) 0
   light *(Arnold* Bakery) . . . . tr.
 oat *(Arnold/Brownberry Bran'nola* Country) . . . . . tr.
 oat bran *(Awrey's)* 0
 oatmeal, light *(Arnold* Bakery) . . . . tr.
 orange raisin *(Brownberry)* . . . . tr.
 pita, all varieties *(Sahara)* 0
 pumpernickel *(Arnold)* 0
 raisin bran *(Brownberry)* 0
 raisin cinnamon or raisin walnut *(Brownberry)* . . . . tr.
 rye:
   (Braun's Old Allegheny) 0
   all varieties *(Beefsteak)* 0
   all varieties *(Brownberry* Natural) 0
   dill *(Arnold)* 0
 Jewish, seeded or seedless *(Levy's)* 0
 sourdough *(DiCarlo)* 0
 sourdough, French *(Boudin)* 0
 wheat:
   (Brownberry Hearth/Natural) 0
   (Fresh & Natural) 0
   (Home Pride Stoneground) 0

Bread, wheat *(cont.)*
    all varieties *(Arnold)* . . . .   tr.
    all varieties *(Beefsteak)*   0
    apple honey *(Brownberry)*   0
    hearty *(Brownberry Bran'nola)* . . . .   tr.
    soft *(Brownberry)* . . . .   tr.
  white, all varieties *(Arnold/Brownberry)* . . . .   tr.

Bread, brown and serve:
    (du Jour Austrian/French), 1 slice   0
    Italian *(Pepperidge Farm),* 1 oz.   0

Bread, brown, canned:
    (S&W New England)   0
    plain or raisin *(B&M/Friends)*   0

Bread dough:
    frozen, all varieties *(Bridgford),* 1 oz.   0
    frozen, white *(Rich's),* 2 slices   0
    refrigerated, all varieties *(Pillsbury/Pipin' Hot)*   0

Bread crumbs:
    plain or Italian style *(Devonsheer),* 1 oz.   0
    plain or Italian style *(Progresso),* 2 tbsp.   0

Breadfruit:
    fresh   0

Breadfruit seeds:
    all varieties, raw, boiled, or roasted   0

Breading mix:
    (Golden Dipt)   0

Breadsticks, refrigerated:
    soft *(Pillsbury),* 1 piece   0
    soft *(Roman Meal),* 1 piece   0

Breakfast strips, see "Bacon, substitute"

The Cholesterol Content of Food

Broad beans:
all varieties, raw, boiled, dried, or canned 0

Broccoli:
fresh or frozen, w/out sauce 0
frozen, in butter sauce:
  (Green Giant One Serving), 4.5 oz. 5
  spears *(Birds Eye* Combinations), 3.3 oz. 5
  spears *(Green Giant)*, 1/2 cup 5
frozen, in cheese sauce:
  (Birds Eye Combinations), 5 oz. 10
  (Stokely Singles), 4 oz. 15
  cuts *(Green Giant* One Serving), 5 oz. 5
  cheese-flavored *(Green Giant)*, 1/2 cup 2

Broccoli combinations, frozen:
all combinations, w/out sauce 0
carrots and rotini, w/cheese sauce *(Green Giant*
  One Serving), 5.5 oz. 5
cauliflower and carrots, w/butter sauce:
  (Birds Eye Combinations), 3.3 oz. 5
  (Green Giant), 1/2 cup 5
cauliflower and carrots, w/cheese sauce:
  (Birds Eye Combinations), 4.5 oz. 5
  (Birds Eye For One), 5 oz. 5
  (Green Giant One Serving), 5 oz. 5
  baby carrots *(Stokely Singles)*, 4 oz. 15
  cheese-flavored sauce *(Green Giant)*, 1/2 cup . . . 2

Broth, see "Bouillon" and "Soup"

Brown gravy mix:
(Hain) 0
(Pillsbury) 0

Brownie, 1 piece or serving:
Dutch chocolate *(Awrey's* Cake), 1/16 cake 35
fudge:
  (Little Debbie), 3 oz. . . . . <1

Brownie, fudge *(cont.)*
    nut *(Awrey's* Sheet Cake), 1.25 oz. 25
    nut, iced *(Awrey's* Sheet Cake), 2.5 oz. 40
    frozen, chocolate *(Weight Watchers)*, 1.25 oz. 5
    frozen, hot fudge *(Pepperidge Farm* Newport) 80

Brownie mix*:
    all varieties *(Betty Crocker)*, 1 piece 10
    all varieties *(Betty Crocker MicroRave)*, 1 piece . . . 0

Browning sauce:
    (Gravymaster) 0

Brussels sprouts:
    fresh or frozen, w/out sauce 0
    frozen, in butter sauce:
      (Green Giant), 1/2 cup 5
      (Stokely Singles), 4 oz. 5
    frozen, w/cheese sauce, baby *(Birds Eye*
      Combinations), 4.5 oz. 5
    frozen, w/cauliflower and carrots *(Birds Eye* Farm
      Fresh), 4 oz. 0

Buckwheat:
    whole-grain or flour 0

Buckwheat groats:
    raw or roasted 0

Bulgur (see also "Tabbouleh mix"):
    dry or cooked 0

Bun, sweet (see also "Roll, sweet"):
    honey, glazed *(Hostess Breakfast Bake Shop)* 15
    honey, iced *(Hostess Breakfast Bake Shop)* 20

Burbot, meat only:
    raw, 1 lb. 270
    raw, 1 oz. 17

Burdock root:

fresh, raw or boiled 0

Burger King, 1 serving:

bagel, 3.2 oz. 29

bagel, w/cream cheese, 4.2 oz. 58

bagel sandwich:

    egg and cheese, 5.7 oz. 247

    bacon, egg, cheese, 6 oz. 252

    ham, egg, cheese, 6.9 oz. 266

    sausage, egg, cheese, 7.4 oz. 293

biscuit, 3.3 oz. 2

biscuit sandwich:

    bacon, 3.6 oz. 8

    bacon and egg, 5.6 oz. 213

    sausage, 4.5 oz. 33

    sausage and egg, 6.5 oz. 238

croissant, 1.4 oz. 4

Croissan'wich:

    egg and cheese, 3.9 oz. 222

    bacon, egg, cheese, 4.2 oz. 227

    ham, egg, cheese, 5.1 oz. 241

    sausage, egg, cheese, 5.6 oz. 268

danish pastry, 4 oz.:

    apple cinnamon 19

    cheese 7

    cinnamon raisin 15

french toast sticks, 5 oz. 80

mini muffins:

    blueberry, 3.4 oz. 72

    lemon-poppyseed, 3 oz. 72

    raisin oat bran, 3.7 oz. 0

scrambled egg platter:

    7.4 oz. 365

    w/bacon, 7.8 oz. 373

    w/sausage, 9.2 oz. 412

Tater Tenders, 2.5 oz. 0

Burger King *(cont.)*
burgers and sandwiches:

BK Broiler chicken sandwich, 5.9 oz.	53
bacon double cheeseburger, 5.6 oz.	105
bacon double cheeseburger deluxe, 6.9 oz.	111
barbecue bacon double cheeseburger, 6.1 oz.	105
Burger Buddies, 4.6 oz.	52
cheeseburger, 4.3 oz.	50
cheeseburger, double, 6.1 oz.	100
cheeseburger deluxe, 5.3 oz.	56
chicken sandwich, 8.1 oz.	82
Chicken Tenders, 3.2 oz.	46
hamburger, 3.8 oz.	37
hamburger deluxe, 4.9 oz.	43
mushroom-Swiss double cheeseburger, 6.2 oz.	95
Ocean Catch fish fillet, 6.8 oz.	57
Whopper, 9.5 oz.	90
Whopper, w/cheese, 10.4 oz.	115
Whopper, double, 12.4 oz.	169
Whopper, double, w/cheese, 13.2 oz.	194

salads, w/out dressing:

chef, 9.6 oz.	103
chicken, chunky, 9.1 oz.	49
garden, 7.9 oz.	15
side, 4.8 oz.	0

salad dressings, *Newman's Own,* 1 pkt.:

bleu cheese	58
French or olive oil and vinegar	0
light Italian, reduced calorie	0
ranch	20
Thousand Island	36

sauces and sandwich condiments:

BK Broiler sauce, .5 oz.	7
bacon bits, .1 oz.	5
Bull's-Eye barbecue sauce, .5 oz.	0
cheese, American, processed, .9 oz.	25
cheese, Swiss, processed, .9 oz.	20
cream cheese, 1 oz.	28

dipping sauces, all varieties, 1 oz. 0
mayonnaise, 1 oz. 16
mushroom topping, .8 oz. 0
tartar sauce, 1 oz. 20
side orders:
  french fries, medium, 4.1 oz. 0
  onion rings, 3.4 oz. 0
desserts:
  apple pie, 4.4 oz. 4
  chocolate shake, 10 oz. 31
  strawberry shake (syrup added), 11 oz. 33
  vanilla shake, 10 oz. 33

"Burger," vegetarian:
canned *(Worthington Vegetarian Burger)* 0
frozen *(Morningstar Farms FriPats/Grillers)* 0
mix*:
  (Love Natural Foods Loveburger) 0
  (Worthington Granburger) 0
  all varieties *(Nature's Burger)* 0

Burrito, frozen (see also "Burrito entree"):
(Patio Britos), 3.63 oz. 15
beef, nacho *(Patio Britos),* 3.63 oz. 25
beef and bean, medium *(Old El Paso),* 1 piece . . . 29
cheese, nacho *(Patio Britos),* 3.63 oz. 20
chicken, spicy *(Patio Britos),* 3.63 oz. 25
chili, green or red *(Patio Britos),* 3.63 oz. 15

Burrito entrée, frozen:
chicken *(Weight Watchers),* 7.62 oz. 60

Burrito mix*:
(Old El Paso Dinner), 1 burrito 23

Burrito seasoning mix:
(Lawry's) 0

Butter, salted or unsalted:
  regular:
    1 stick or 4 oz. 248
    1 tbsp. 31
    1 tsp. 10
    1 pat (90 per lb.) 11
  whipped:
    1/2 cup or 1 stick 165
    1 tbsp. 20
    1 tsp. 7
    1 pat (120 per lb.) 8

Butter oil:
  1 tbsp. 33

Butterbur:
  fresh or canned, plain 0

Butterfish, meat only:
  raw, 1 lb. 295
  raw, 1 oz. 18

Buttermilk, see "Milk" and "Milk, dry"

Butternut:
  dried 0

Butternut squash:
  fresh or frozen 0

Butterscotch topping:
  (Kraft) 0
  flavor *(Smucker's)* 0

C

Food and Measure	Cholesterol (mgs.)
Cabbage:	
all varieties, fresh or canned	0
Cabbage, stuffed, frozen:	
w/meat, in tomato sauce *(Lean Cuisine)*, 10.75 oz.	55
Cajun seasoning:	
(Tone's)	0
Cake:	
apple streusel *(Awrey's)*, 2″ × 2″ piece	15
banana, iced *(Awrey's)*, 2″ × 2″ piece	20
Black Forest torte *(Awrey's)*, 1/14 cake	50
carrot, iced, supreme *(Awrey's)*, 2″ × 2″ piece	25

Cake *(cont.)*

carrot, iced, 3-layer *(Awrey's)*, 1/12 cake	45
chocolate:	
double, iced *(Awrey's)*, 2″ × 2″ piece	15
double, 2-layer or 3-layer *(Awrey's)*, 1/12 cake . .	35
double torte *(Awrey's)*, 1/14 cake	35
German, iced *(Awrey's)*, 2″ × 2″ piece	20
German, 3-layer *(Awrey's)*, 1/12 cake	40
milk, yellow, 2-layer *(Awrey's)*, 1/12 cake	50
white iced, 2-layer *(Awrey's)*, 1/12 cake	40
coconut, butter cream *(Awrey's)*, 2″ × 2″ piece . . .	25
coconut, yellow, 3-layer *(Awrey's)*, 1/12 cake	50
coffee, caramel nut *(Awrey's)*, 1/12 cake	5
coffee, long John *(Awrey's)*, 1/12 cake	10
devil's food, iced *(Awrey's)*, 2″ × 2″ piece	25
lemon, 3-layer *(Awrey's)*, 1/12 cake	45
lemon, yellow, 2-layer *(Awrey's)*, 1/12 cake	45
Neapolitan torte *(Awrey's)*, 1/14 cake	55
orange, iced, frosty *(Awrey's)*, 2″ × 2″ piece	20
orange, three-layer *(Awrey's)*, 1/12 cake	35
peanut butter, torte *(Awrey's)*, 1/14 cake	40
pistachio, torte *(Awrey's)*, 1/14 cake	35
pound *(Drake's)*, 1/10 cake	25
pound, golden *(Awrey's)*, 1/14 loaf	20
raisin spice, iced *(Awrey's)*, 2″ × 2″ piece	20
raspberry nut *(Awrey's)*, 1/16 cake	30
sponge *(Awrey's)*, 2″ × 2″ piece	15
strawberry supreme, torte *(Awrey's)*, 1/14 cake . . .	45
walnut, torte *(Awrey's)*, 1/14 cake	30
yellow, iced *(Awrey's)*, 2″ × 2″ piece	25

Cake, frozen:

all varieties *(Sara Lee Free & Light)*	0
Boston cream *(Pepperidge Farm* Supreme),	
1/4 cake	50
Boston cream *(Weight Watchers)*, 3 oz.	5
carrot:	
(Weight Watchers), 3 oz.	5

cream cheese iced *(Pepperidge Farm* Old
  Fashioned), 1/8 cake 15
single layer, iced *(Sara Lee)*, 1/8 cake 25
cheesecake:
  (Weight Watchers), 3.9 oz. 20
  brownie *(Weight Watchers)*, 3.5 oz. 10
  French *(Sara Lee* Classics), 1/8 cake 20
  strawberry *(Weight Watchers)*, 3.9 oz. 20
  strawberry, French *(Sara Lee)*, 1/8 cake 20
cheesecake, nondairy, all varieties *(Tofutti Better
  than Cheesecake)*, 2 oz. 0
cherries and cream *(Weight Watchers)*, 3 oz. 5
chocolate:
  (Pepperidge Farm Supreme), 1/4 cake 25
  (Weight Watchers), 2.5 oz. 5
  double, three layer *(Sara Lee)*, 1/8 cake 20
  fudge, double *(Weight Watchers)*, 2.75 oz. 5
  fudge layer, fudge stripe, or German layer
    (Pepperidge Farm), 1/10 cake 20
  German *(Weight Watchers)*, 2.5 oz. 5
  mousse *(Sara Lee* Classics), 1/8 cake 20
coconut layer *(Pepperidge Farm)*, 1/10 cake 20
coffee, cinnamon streusel *(Weight Watchers)*,
  2.25 oz. or 1/2 pkg. 5
devil's food layer *(Pepperidge Farm)*, 1/10 cake . . . 20
golden layer *(Pepperidge Farm)*, 1/10 cake 20
lemon coconut *(Pepperidge Farm* Supreme),
  1/4 cake 30
lemon cream or pineapple cream *(Pepperidge Farm*
  Supreme), 1/12 cake 20
pound *(Pepperidge Farm* Old Fashioned
  Cholesterol Free), 1/10 cake 0
strawberry cream or strawberry stripe layer
  (Pepperidge Farm Supreme), 1/12 cake 20
vanilla layer *(Pepperidge Farm)*, 1/10 cake 20

Cake, refrigerated:
coffee, all varieties *(Pillsbury)* 0

Cake, snack, 1 piece:

apple bar, baked *(Sunbelt)*	<1
apple delight or spice *(Little Debbie)*	<1
apple spice *(Hostess Light)*	0
banana *(Hostess Suzy Q's)*	20
banana *(Hostess Twinkies)*	20
banana twins *(Little Debbie)*	<1
brownie, see "Brownie"	
caramel peanut filled *(Little Debbie Peanut Cluster)*	<1
chocolate:	
(Hostess Choco Bliss/Ding Dongs)	5
(Hostess Choco-Diles)	20
(Hostess Ho Hos)	10
(Hostess Suzy Q's)	15
(Little Debbie)	<1
(Little Debbie Choco-Cake/Choco-Jel)	<1
cream filled *(Drake's Devil Dog/Ring Ding)*	0
fudge crispy or fudge round *(Little Debbie)*	<1
mint, cream-filled *(Drake's Ring Ding)*	0
roll, cream-filled *(Drake's Yodel)*	5
roll, cream-filled, Swiss *(Drake's)*	15
slices or twins *(Little Debbie)*	<1
w/vanilla pudding *(Hostess Light)*	0
chocolate chip *(Little Debbie)*	<1
coconut covered *(Hostess Sno Balls)*	2
coconut crunch *(Little Debbie)*	<2
coffee:	
(Drake's Jr.)	10
(Drake's Small)	15
(Little Debbie)	<1
cinnamon crumb *(Drake's)*	10
crumb cake *(Hostess)*	9
crumb cake *(Hostess Light)*	0
cupcake:	
chocolate *(Hostess)*	5
chocolate, cream filled *(Drake's Yankee Doodle)*	0
chocolate, creme filled *(Hostess Light)*	0
golden, cream filled *(Drake's Sunny Doodle)*	10

orange *(Hostess)*	10
dessert cup *(Little Debbie)*	<1
devil's food *(Little Debbie Devil Cremes)*	<1
devil's food *(Little Debbie Devil Squares)*	<1
(Drake's Funny Bone)	0
(Drake's Zoinks)	10
fancy *(Little Debbie)*	<1
fig *(Little Debbie Figaroos)*	<1
golden cremes *(Little Debbie)*	<1
(Hostess Lil' Angels)	2
(Hostess Tiger Tails)	25
(Hostess Twinkies)	20
(Hostess Twinkies Light)	0
jelly roll or lemon stix *(Little Debbie)*	<1
(Little Debbie Caravella/Doodle Dandies)	<1
marshmallow supreme *(Little Debbie)*	<1
mint wafer, chocolate coated *(Little Debbie Mint Sprints)*	<1
peanut butter bar, wafer, or jelly sandwich *(Little Debbie)*	<1
pecan twins *(Little Debbie)*	<1
pie, see "Pie, snack"	
strawberry *(Hostess Twinkies Fruit N Creme)*	20
Swiss roll or vanilla *(Little Debbie)*	<1

Cake, snack, frozen, 1 piece or serving:

apple crisp *(Sara Lee Lights)*	5
apple'n spice bake *(Pepperidge Farm Dessert Lights)*	10
Black Forest *(Sara Lee Lights)*	10
carrot:	
(Pepperidge Farm Classic)	50
(Sara Lee)	10
(Sara Lee Lights)	5
cheesecake:	
French *(Sara Lee Lights)*	15
strawberry *(Pepperidge Farm Manhattan)*	150
strawberry, French *(Sara Lee Lights)*	5

Cake, snack, frozen *(cont.)*
  cherries supreme *(Pepperidge Farm Dessert Lights)*   80
  chocolate:
    double *(Pepperidge Farm Classic)* 35
    double *(Sara Lee Lights)* 10
    fudge *(Pepperidge Farm Classic)* 40
    German *(Pepperidge Farm Classic)* 45
  chocolate mousse:
    (Pepperidge Farm Dessert Lights)   5
    (Pepperidge Farm San Francisco) 150
    (Sara Lee) 15
    (Sara Lee Lights) 10
  coconut *(Pepperidge Farm Classic)* 20
  lemon cream *(Sara Lee Lights)* 10
  lemon supreme *(Pepperidge Farm Dessert Lights)*   50
  peach parfait *(Pepperidge Farm Dessert Lights)* . . 10
  raspberry-vanilla swirl *(Pepperidge Farm Dessert Lights)* 15
  strawberry shortcake *(Pepperidge Farm Dessert Lights)* 70
  vanilla fudge swirl *(Pepperidge Farm Classic)* 35

Cake frosting, see "Frosting"

Cake mix*, 1/12 cake or pkg., except as noted:
  angel food, all varieties *(Betty Crocker)*   0
  angel food *(Duncan Hines)*   0
  apple cinnamon, butter pecan, or carrot *(Betty Crocker SuperMoist)* 55
  apple streusel *(Betty Crocker MicroRave)*, 1/6 cake   45
  cheesecake, no bake:
    (Jell-O/Jell-O New York Style), 1/8 cake 30
    lemon *(Jell-O)*, 1/8 cake 25
  cherry chip *(Betty Crocker SuperMoist)*   0
  chocolate:
    butter *(Betty Crocker SuperMoist)* 75

fudge, German, or milk *(Betty Crocker SuperMoist)* 55

fudge, w/vanilla frosting *(Betty Crocker MicroRave)*, 1/6 cake 35

German, w/coconut pecan frosting *(Betty Crocker MicroRave)*, 1/6 cake 35

chocolate chip, all varieties *(Betty Crocker SuperMoist)* 55

cinnamon pecan streusel *(Betty Crocker MicroRave)*, 1/6 cake 45

coffee *(Aunt Jemima Easy)*, 1 serving 1

devil's food *(Betty Crocker SuperMoist)* 55

devil's food, w/chocolate frosting *(Betty Crocker MicroRave)*, 1/6 cake 35

gingerbread *(Betty Crocker Classic)*, 1/9 cake 30

lemon or marble *(Betty Crocker SuperMoist)* 55

lemon, w/lemon frosting *(Pillsbury MicroRave)*, 1/6 cake 45

pineapple upside-down *(Betty Crocker Classic)*, 1/9 cake 40

pound *(Martha White)*, 1/10 cake 8

pound, golden *(Betty Crocker Classic)* 35

rainbow chip, sour cream chocolate, spice, yellow, vanilla *(Betty Crocker SuperMoist)* 55

sour cream white *(Betty Crocker SuperMoist)* 0

vanilla, golden, w/rainbow chip frosting *(Betty Crocker MicroRave)*, 1/6 cake 35

white *(Betty Crocker SuperMoist)* 0

yellow, butter *(Betty Crocker SuperMoist)* 75

yellow, w/chocolate frosting *(Betty Crocker MicroRave)*, 1/6 cake 35

Calves' liver, see "Liver, veal"

Candy:

candy cane *(Brach's)* 0

candy cane *(Spangler)* 0

Candy *(cont.)*
caramel:
  (Caramello), 1.6 oz. 10
  (Kraft) 0
  chocolate-coated *(Rolo)*, 8 pieces 15
chocolate:
  w/almonds *(Hershey's Golden Almond)*, 1.6 oz. 5
  w/almonds *(Hershey's Solitaires)*, 1.6 oz. 5
  chips, see "Chocolate, baking"
  dark, sweet *(Hershey's Special Dark)*, 1.45 oz. . . 0
  milk *(Hershey's)*, 1.55 oz. 10
  milk *(Hershey's Kisses)*, 9 pieces 10
  milk, w/almonds *(Hershey's)*, 1.45 oz. 15
  milk, w/crisps *(Krackel)*, 1.55 oz. 10
  milk, w/peanuts *(Mr. Goodbar)*, 1.75 oz. 15
cinnamon, all varieties *(Brach's)* 0
coconut, chocolate-coated:
  (Mounds), 1.9 oz. 0
  (Sunbelt Macaroo), 2 oz. . . . . <1
  w/almonds *(Almond Joy)*, 1.76 oz. 0
corn, Indian *(Brach's)* 0
cough drops, all varieties 0
cremes, chocolate-coated, all varieties *(Spangler)* 0
fruit flavored, all flavors:
  (Brach's Fruit Bunch) 0
  (Skittles) 0
  chews *(Bonkers!)* 0
  chews *(Starburst)* 0
fudge *(Kraft* Fudgies) 0
fudge, all flavors *(Woodys)*, 1 oz. 5
gum, chewing, all flavors (all brands) 0
hard, all varieties, all flavors *(Life Savers)* 0
(Hot Tamales) 0
jellied and gummed, all varieties 0
(Jolly Joes) 0
lemon drops *(Brach's)* 0
licorice, all varieties (all brands) 0

The Cholesterol Content of Food

lollipop, all flavors:
  (Brach's Pops) 0
  (Life Savers) 0
  (Spangler) 0
  (Tootsie Pop), 1 oz. . . . . tr.
lozenge (Listerine) 0
marshmallow, plain (all brands) 0
mint:
  (Brach's Coolers/Kentucky/Starlight) 0
  (Certs Sugar Free) 0
  (Mint Meltaway) 0
  all flavors (Breath Savers) 0
  butter or party (Kraft) 0
  pattie, chocolate-coated (York Peppermint
    Pattie), 1.5 oz. 0
nougat (Brach's) 0
orange (Brach's Orangettes) 0
peanut, French burnt (Brach's) 0
peanut brittle (Kraft) 0
peanut butter, candy-coated (Reese's Pieces),
  1.85 oz. 5
peanut butter cup, chocolate-coated (Reese's),
  1.8 oz. 10
popcorn, caramel-coated (Orville Redenbacher) . . 0
popcorn, caramel-coated, w/peanuts (Cracker
  Jack) 0
raspberry filled (Brach's) 0
rock (Brach's Cut Rock) 0
(Rolaids) 0
sour balls (Brach's) 0
spice (Brach's Spicettes) 0
straws, mint-filled (Brach's) 0
taffy, all flavors (Brach's Salt Water Taffy) 0
taffy, all flavors, chews (Beich's Laffy Taffy) 0
toffee:
  (Brach's) 0
  (Callard & Bowser) 0
  (Skor), 1.4 oz. 25

Candy *(cont.)*
  (Tootsie Roll), 1 oz. . . . .   tr.
  wafer, all flavors *(Necco)*   0
  wafer bar, chocolate-coated *(Kit Kat),* 1.63 oz. . . .   10

Cane syrup:
  1 tbsp.   0

Cannelloni dinner, frozen:
  chicken *(Le Menu* LightStyle), 1.25 oz.   65

Cannelloni entrée, frozen:
  beef and pork, w/Mornay sauce *(Lean Cuisine),*
    $9^5/_8$ oz.   45
  cheese *(Dining Lite),* 9 oz.   70
  cheese, w/tomato sauce *(Lean Cuisine),* $9^1/_8$ oz. . .   35

Cantaloupe:
  fresh   0

Capon, see "Chicken"

Carambola:
  fresh   0

Caramel, see "Candy"

Caramel topping:
  (Kraft)   0
  all varieties *(Smucker's)*   0

Caraway seeds:
  dried   0

Cardamom:
  ground or seed   0

The Cholesterol Content of Food

Cardoon:
fresh, raw or boiled 0

Carissa:
fresh 0

Carl's Jr., 1 serving:
breakfast:
  bacon, 2 strips 8
  English muffin, w/margarine 0
  French toast dips, w/out syrup 54
  hash brown nuggets 10
  hot cakes w/margarine, w/out syrup 15
  sausage, 1 patty 25
  scrambled eggs 245
  Sunrise Sandwich, w/bacon 120
  Sunrise Sandwich, w/sausage 165
sandwiches:
  California Roast Beef 'n Swiss 130
  Charbroiler BBQ Chicken Sandwich 50
  Charbroiler Chicken Club Sandwich 85
  Country Fried Steak 45
  Double Western Bacon Cheeseburger 145
  Famous Star Hamburger 45
  fish fillet 90
  Happy Star hamburger 45
  Old Time Star hamburger 80
  Super Star hamburger 125
  Western Bacon Cheeseburger 105
potatoes:
  bacon and cheese 45
  broccoli and cheese 10
  cheese 40
  Fiesta 40
  sour cream and chive 10
salad-to-go:
  chef 63
  chicken 83

Carl's Jr., salad-to-go *(cont.)*
garden	7
taco	99

salad dressing, 1 oz.:
blue cheese	18
French, reduced calorie	0
house	10
Italian	0
Thousand Island	5

side dishes:
french fries, regular	15
onion rings	10
zucchini	10

soup, 6.6 oz.:
Boston clam chowder	22
broccoli, cream of	22
chicken noodle	14
Lumber Jack Mix vegetable	3

bakery products:
blueberry muffin	34
bran muffin	50
brownie, fudge	tr.
chocolate chip cookie	3
cinnamon roll or danish (varieties)	tr.

shake, regular	17

Carob drink mix:
powder	0

Carob flour:
all varieties	0

Carp, meat only:
raw, 1 lb.	298
raw, 1 oz.	19
baked, broiled, or microwaved, 4 oz.	95

Carrot:
fresh, canned, or frozen, w/out sauce   0

Carrot chips:
all varieties *(Hain)*   0

Carrot juice:
fresh or canned   0

Casaba:
fresh   0

Cashew:
all varieties   0

Cashew butter:
all varieties (all brands)   0

Cassava:
fresh   0

Catfish:
fresh, channel, meat only, 1 lb.   263
fresh, channel, meat only, raw, 1 oz.   16
frozen *(Delta Pride),* 4 oz.   62

Catjang:
dried or cooked   0

Catsup:
(all brands)   0

Cauliflower:
fresh or frozen, w/out sauce   0
frozen, in cheese sauce:
   (Birds Eye Combinations), 5 oz.   10
   (Stokely Singles), 4 oz.   15
   cheddar *(The Budget Gourmet),* 5 oz.   25

Caviar, granular:
  black or red, 1 oz. 165
  black or red, 1 tbsp. 94

Celeriac:
  fresh 0

Celery:
  fresh or dried 0

Celery seed or salt:
  (all brands) 0

Cellophane noodles, see "Noodle, Chinese"

Celtus:
  fresh 0

Cereal, ready-to-eat, 1 oz., except as noted:
  bran:
    (Bran Buds) 0
    (Bran Chex) 0
    (Nabisco 100% Bran) 0
    (Quaker Crunchy Bran) 0
    all varieties *(All Bran)* 0
    all varieties *(Fruitful Bran)* 0
    all varieties *(Kellogg's)* 0
    all varieties *(Post)* 0
    w/fruit and nuts *(Müeslix)* 0
  corn:
    (Corn Chex) 0
    (Corn Pops) 0
    (Kellogg's Corn Flakes) 0
    (Kellogg's Frosted Flakes) 0
    (Nutri · Grain) 0
    (Post Toasties) 0
    (Total Corn Flakes) 0

The Cholesterol Content of Food

granola:
- (*C.W. Post* Hearty) 0
- all varieties (*Sun Country* 100% Natural) 0
- banana almond or fruit and nut (*Sunbelt*) ..... <1

mixed grain and natural style:
- (*Almond Delight*) 0
- (*Crispix*) 0
- (*Crunchy Nut Oh!s*) 0
- (*Double Chex*) 0
- (*Fiber One*) 0
- (*Honey Graham Chex*) 0
- (*Honey Graham Oh!s*) 0
- (*Product 19*) 0
- (*Special K*) 0
- (*Sunflakes MultiGrain*) 0
- all varieties (*Fruit & Fibre*) 0
- all varieties (*Grape-Nuts*) 0
- all varieties (*Heartland*) 0
- all varieties (*Honey Bunches of Oats*) 0
- all varieties (*Just Right*) 0
- all varieties (*Müeslix*) 0
- all varieties (*Nature Valley*) 0
- all varieties (*Nutri·Grain*) 0
- all varieties (*Quaker* 100% Natural) 0
- all varieties (*Ralston Muesli*) 0
- w/apples and raisins (*Apple Raisin Crisp*) 0
- w/raisins and almonds (*Nutrific*) 0

oat:
- (*Alpha-Bits*) 0
- (*Oat Chex*) 0
- (*Quaker Oat Squares*) 0
- all varieties (*Cheerios*) 0
- all varieties (*Life*) 0
- toasted (*Nature Valley*) 0

oat bran:
- (*Cracklin' Oat Bran*) 0
- (*Post* Oat Flakes) 0
- all varieties (*Common Sense*) 0

Cereal, ready-to-eat, oat bran *(cont.)*

    w/raisins *(General Mills)*, 1.5 oz.   0

    w/raisins *(Raisin Oat Bran Options)*, 1.45 oz. . . .   0

  rice:

    (Rice Chex)   0

    all varieties *(Kellogg's)*   0

    puffed *(Quaker)*, .5 oz., approx. 1 cup   0

  wheat:

    (Wheat Chex)   0

    (Wheaties)   0

    all varieties *(Nutri·Grain)*   0

    all varieties *(Total)*   0

    puffed *(Quaker)*, .5 oz. or 1 cup   0

    w/raisins *(General Mills* Raisin Nut Bran)   0

  wheat, shredded:

    (Nutri·Grain)   0

    (Quaker), 2 pieces   0

    (Sunshine), 2 pieces   0

    all varieties *(Nabisco)*   0

    all varieties *(S.W. Graham)*   0

    bite size *(Sunshine)*, 2/3 cup   0

    regular or bite size *(Frosted Mini-Wheats)*   0

Cereal, cooking, uncooked, all varieties:

  (Cream of Wheat)   0

  (H-O Brand)   0

  (Maypo 30 Second)   0

  (Quaker/Mother's)   0

  (Roman Meal)   0

  (Total)   0

  (Wheatena)   0

  (Wholesome 'N Hearty)   0

Cereal beverage, see "Coffee, substitute"

Chard, Swiss, see "Swiss chard"

Chayote:
raw or cooked 0

Cheese (see also "Cheese food"), 1 oz., except as
noted:
all varieties, except mozzarella *(Kraft Light Naturals)* 20
American, processed:
   (Kraft Deluxe loaf or slices) 25
   (Land O'Lakes) 25
   hot pepper *(Sargento)* 27
   sharp *(Old English* loaf or slices) 30
babybel *(Laughing Cow)* 22
(Bel Paese Domestic Traditional) 20
(Bel Paese Imported) 22
(Bel Paese Lite) 16
(Bel Paese Medallion) 18
blue:
   (Dorman's Danablu 50%) 23
   (Dorman's Danablu 60%) 31
   (Sargento) 21
   blue castello or saga *(Dorman's* 70%) 29
blue or brick *(Kraft)* 30
bonbel *(Laughing Cow)* 24
bonbino *(Laughing Cow)* 27
brick *(Land O'Lakes)* 25
Brie *(Dorman's)* 20
Brie or cajun *(Sargento)* 28
Camembert:
   (Dorman's 45%) 17
   (Dorman's 50%) 23
   (Sargento) 20
cheddar:
   (Kraft) 30
   (Land O'Lakes) 30
   (Laughing Cow) 28
   (Sargento) 30
   reduced fat *(Dorman's* Low Sodium) 20
   sharp or extra sharp *(Axelrod)* 30

Cheese, cheddar *(cont.)*

sharp, slicing *(Boar's Head)*	18
sharp, white *(Cracker Barrel Light* Natural)	20
Vermont *(Churny)*	30
Cheshire	29
colby *(Kraft)*	30
colby *(Land O'Lakes)*	25
colby or colby jack *(Sargento)*	27
cottage cheese, creamed:	
(Darigold), 4 oz.	17
(Friendship California Style), 1/2 cup	17
(Knudsen Large or Small Curd), 4 oz.	20
garden salad or pineapple *(Bison)*, 1/2 cup	15
w/peach *(Crowley)*, 1/2 cup	10
w/pineapple *(Friendship)*, 1/2 cup	17
plain or chive *(Bison)*, 1/2 cup	20
plain or w/pineapple *(Breakstone's)*, 4 oz.	25
plain or w/pineapple *(Crowley)*, 1/2 cup	15
cottage cheese, dry curd *(Breakstone's)*, 4 oz. . . .	10
cottage cheese, lowfat:	
2% *(Breakstone's/Sealtest)*, 4 oz.	15
2% *(Darigold* Trim), 4 oz.	17
2% *(Knudsen)*, 4 oz.	15
1% *(Crowley)*, 1/2 cup	5
1% *(Friendship)*, 1/2 cup	5
all varieties *(Light N' Lively* 1%), 4 oz.	10
w/apple, spiced *(Knudsen* 2%), 6 oz.	15
w/fruit cocktail, Mandarin orange, or pear,	
(Knudsen 2%), 4 oz.	10
w/peach, pineapple, or strawberry *(Knudsen*	
2%), 6 oz.	15
w/pineapple *(Crowley* 1%), 1/2 cup	5
pot style *(Friendship* 2%), 1/2 cup	9
cottage cheese, nonfat *(Knudsen)*, 4 oz.	5
cream cheese:	
(Crowley)	30
(Dorman's 65%)	26
(Dorman's 70%)	30

(Philadelphia Brand)	30
w/chives or pimiento *(Philadelphia Brand)*	30
cream cheese, soft:	
(Friendship)	31
(Philadelphia Brand)	30
w/chives and onion *(Philadelphia Brand)*	30
w/herbs and garlic, olives and pimiento, or	
pineapple *(Philadelphia Brand)*	25
w/smoked salmon *(Philadelphia Brand)*	25
w/strawberries *(Philadelphia Brand)*	20
cream cheese, whipped:	
all varieties, except w/onions *(Philadelphia Brand)*	30
w/onions *(Philadelphia Brand)*	25
danbo *(Dorman's 20%)*	9
danbo *(Dorman's 45%)*	23
(Dorman's Crema Dania 70%)	29
Edam:	
(Dorman's 45%)	21
(Kaukauna)	25
(Kraft)	20
(Land O'Lakes)	25
(Laughing Cow)	26
(Sargento)	25
farmer:	
(Friendship), 4 oz.	40
(Kaukauna)	25
(May-Bud)	20
(Sargento)	26
feta *(Churny* Natural)	25
feta *(Sargento)*	25
fontina *(Sargento)*	33
Gouda:	
(Kraft)	30
(Land O'Lakes)	30
(Laughing Cow)	28
(Sargento)	32
plain or w/caraway seed *(Kaukauna)*	30
w/hickory smoke flavor *(Kaukauna)*	25

Cheese, Gouda *(cont.)*
  mini *(Laughing Cow)*, 3/4 oz. 21
Gruyère 31
havarti:
  (Casino) 35
  (Dorman's 45%) 21
  (Dorman's 60%) 31
  (Sargento) 31
Italian style, grated *(Sargento)* 26
Jarlsberg *(Norseland)* 18
Limburger *(Mohawk Valley Little Gem)* 25
Limburger *(Sargento)* 26
mascarpone *(Galbani Imported)* 39
Monterey Jack:
  (Alpine Lace Monti-Jack-Lo) 15
  (Darigold) 25
  (Kaukauna) 25
  (Sargento) 25
  plain, w/caraway seeds, or jalapeño *(Kraft)* 30
  plain or w/jalapeños *(Axelrod)* 30
mozzarella:
  (Polly-O Lite) 15
  fresh *(Polly-O Fior di Latte)* 20
  whole milk *(Crowley)* 25
  whole milk *(Frigo)* 15
  whole milk *(Polly-O)* 20
  whole milk *(Sargento)* 25
  low moisture *(Kraft)* 20
  part skim *(Alpine Lace)* 15
  part skim *(Crowley)* 15
  part skim *(Dorman's Low Sodium)* 15
  part skim *(Frigo)* 10
  part skim *(Polly-O)* 15
  part skim *(Sargento)* 15
  part skim, low moisture *(Kraft)* 15
  part skim, w/jalapeño pepper *(Kraft)* 20
  reduced fat *(Dorman's Low Sodium)* 17
  reduced fat *(Kraft Light Naturals)* 15

Muenster:
(Alpine Lace) 30
(Dorman's 50%) 24
(Kaukauna) 25
(Land O'Lakes) 25
red rind *(Sargento)* 27
reduced fat *(Dorman's* Low Sodium) 18
Neufchâtel:
(Philadelphia Brand Light) 25
garlic and herb or vegetable *(Kaukauna)* 25
Parmesan:
(Kraft) 20
fresh *(Sargento)* 19
grated *(Kraft)* 30
grated *(Polly-O)* 20
grated *(Progresso)*, 1 tbsp. 4
grated *(Sargento)* 22
Reggiano *(Galbani* Imported) 21
Parmesan and Romano, grated *(Sargento)* 24
pimiento, processed *(Kraft* Deluxe) 25
pizza, shredded *(Frigo)* 20
pizza, shredded, low fat *(Frigo)* 10
Port du Salut 35
primavera *(Bel Paese* Lite) 14
provolone:
(Alpine Lace Provo-Lo) 15
(Kraft) 25
(Land O'Lakes) 20
(Sargento) 20
queso blanco *(Sargento)* 27
queso de papa *(Sargento)* 30
ricotta, 2 oz., except as noted:
(Polly-O Lite) 15
(Sargento), 1 oz. 13
(Sargento Lite), 1 oz. 4
whole milk, 1/2 cup 63
whole milk *(Crowley)* 25
whole milk or part skim *(Polly-O)* 20

Cheese, ricotta *(cont.)*
    part skim *(Crowley)*   15
    lowfat *(Frigo)*, 1 oz.   5
  Romano:
    (Kraft Natural)   20
    (Sargento)   29
    grated *(Kraft)*   30
    grated *(Polly-O)*   30
    grated *(Progresso)*, 1 tbsp.   6
  Roquefort, sheep's milk   26
  smoked *(Sargento Smokestick)*   24
  string:
    (Polly-O Stick)   15
    (Sargento)   15
    low moisture *(Kraft)*   20
  Swiss:
    (Alpine Lace Swiss-Lo)   20
    (Boar's Head Domestic)   25
    (Casino)   30
    (Dorman's Reduced Fat)   17
    (Kraft Light Naturals)   20
    (Kraft 75% Very Low Sodium)   25
    (Sargento)   26
    baby *(Cracker Barrel* Natural)   25
    Finland *(Sargento)*   26
    processed *(Kraft* Deluxe)   25
    regular or aged *(Kraft)*   25
  taco *(Sargento)*   27
  taco, shredded *(Kraft)*   30
  Tilsit *(Sargento)*   29
  Tybo *(Dorman's* 45%)   23
  Tybo, red wax *(Sargento)*   23

Cheese, imitation and substitute, 1 oz.:
  (Nucoa Heart Beat)   0
  all varieties *(Dorman's* LoChol)   1
  all varieties *(Golden Image)*   5

all varieties, except American, hickory smoke
   (Churny Delicia) 3
American, hickory smoke *(Churny* Delicia) 1
cheddar or mozzarella, imitation *(Frigo)* 0
cheddar or mozzarella, imitation *(Sargento)* 2
cream cheese, imitation, all varieties *(Tofutti Better
   than Cream Cheese)* 0

Cheese danish, frozen:
twist *(Sara Lee),* 1/8 pkg. 15

Cheese dip:
blue or nacho *(Kraft* Premium), 2 tbsp. 10

Cheese food (see also "Cheese product"), 1 oz.:
(Nippy) 20
all varieties:
   (Cracker Barrel) 20
   (Kaukauna Cup) 25
   (Kaukauna Lite) 15
   except white American *(Kraft* Singles) 25
   except onion *(Land O'Lakes)* 20
American:
   (Darigold) 16
   grated *(Kraft)* 25
   white *(Kraft* Singles) 20
cheddar or port wine, cold pack *(Wispride)* 25
w/garlic or jalapeños *(Kraft)* 20
w/jalapeños, hot or mild *(Velveeta* Mexican) 25
onion *(Land O'Lakes)* 15
shredded *(Velveeta)* 20

Cheese-nut ball or log, 1 oz.:
all varieties *(Kaukauna)* 25
ball, sharp cheddar, w/almonds *(Cracker Barrel)* . . 20
log, all varieties *(Cracker Barrel)* 15
log, sharp cheddar or port wine *(Sargento)* 18
log, Swiss almond *(Sargento)* 21

Cheese product (see also "Cheese spread"), 1 oz.:
(Velveeta Light Singles)   15
all varieties *(Kraft Light)*   15
all varieties *(Light N' Lively* Singles)   15
American flavor:
  (Alpine Lace)   20
  (Harvest Moon)   15
  (Kraft Free)   5
cheddar, all varieties *(Spreadery)*   15
cream cheese *(Philadelphia Brand Light)*   10
Mexican w/jalapeños, or nacho *(Spreadery)*   15
Neufchâtel, all varieties, except w/strawberry
  (Spreadery)   20
Neufchâtel, w/strawberry *(Spreadery)*   15
port wine *(Spreadery)*   15
port wine flavor *(Weight Watchers* Diet Snack) . . .   10
sandwich slices *(Lunch Wagon)*   5

Cheese sauce:
nacho *(Kaukauna)*, 1 oz.   8
refrigerated, four cheese *(Contadina Fresh)*, 6 oz.   147

Cheese spread (see also "Cheese"), 1 oz., except
as noted:
(Land O'Lakes Golden Velvet)   15
(Laughing Cow Cheezbits), 1/6 oz.   3
(Micro Melt)   15
all varieties:
  (Cheez Whiz)   20
  (Squeez-A-Snak)   20
  (Velveeta)   20
American, processed *(Kraft)*   15
American, processed, w/pimiento, or sharp
  (Sargento Cracker Snacks)   27
w/bacon *(Kraft)*   20
blue *(Roka)*   20
brick *(Sargento* Cracker Snacks)   25
jalapeño *(Kraft)*   15

jalapeño loaf *(Kraft)* 20
Limburger *(Mohawk Valley)* 20
olive and pimiento, pimiento, or pineapple *(Kraft)* . . 15
sharp *(Old English)* 20
Swiss *(Sargento* Cracker Snacks) 24

Cherimoya:
fresh 0

Cherry:
all varieties, fresh, canned, dried, or frozen 0

Cherry drink or juice:
bottled or mix (all brands) 0

Cherry fruit concentrate:
black *(Hain)* 0

Chervil:
fresh or dried 0

Chestnuts:
all varieties, raw, dried, boiled, or roasted 0

Chicken, fresh, 4 oz., except as noted:
broiler-fryer, fried, flour coated, w/skin:
4 oz. 102
light meat 99
dark meat 104
skin only, 1 oz. 21
broiler-fryer, roasted:
w/skin, 1/2 chicken, 10.5 oz. (15.8 oz. w/bone) . . 263
w/skin 100
meat only 101
meat only, chopped or diced, 1 cup not packed 125
skin only, 1 oz. 24
dark meat w/skin 103
dark meat only 105

Chicken, broiler-fryer, roasted *(cont.)*

light meat w/skin	95
light meat only	96
back, meat w/skin	100
back, meat only	102
breast, meat w/skin	95
breast, meat only	96
drumstick, meat w/skin	103
drumstick, meat only	105
leg, meat w/skin, 4 oz. (5.7 oz. leg w/bone)	105
leg, meat only	107
thigh, meat w/skin	105
thigh, meat only	108
wing, meat w/skin, 1.2 oz. (2.3 oz. wing w/bone)	29
capon, roasted:	
w/skin, 1/2 capon, 1.4 lbs. (2 lbs. w/bone)	549
w/skin	98
roaster, roasted:	
w/skin, 1/2 chicken, 1 lb. (1.5 lbs. w/bone)	365
w/skin	86
stewing, stewed:	
w/skin, 1/2 chicken, 9.2 oz. (13.5 oz. w/bone) . . .	205
w/skin	90
meat only	94
meat only, chopped or diced, 1 cup	117

Chicken, canned:

chunk, white *(Swanson Premium)*, 2 1/2 oz.	35
chunk, white and dark meat *(Swanson)*, 2 1/2 oz. . .	40

"Chicken," vegetarian:

canned or frozen, all varieties *(Worthington)*	0
frozen, all varieties *(Morningstar Farms)*	0

Chicken, luncheon meat and boneless:

breast:	
(Longacre Premium), 1 oz.	20
(Mr. Turkey), 1 oz.	9
hickory smoked *(Louis Rich)*, 1 oz.	14

oven-roasted (*Louis Rich* Deluxe), 1 oz. 14
oven-roasted (*Louis Rich* Thin Sliced), .4-oz.
  slice 6
oven-roasted (*Oscar Mayer*), .4-oz. slice 7
oven-roasted (*Oscar Mayer*), 1 oz. 15
roast (*Oscar Mayer* Thin Sliced), .4-oz. slice . . . 5
smoked (*Eckrich Lite*), 1 oz. 20
smoked (*Oscar Mayer*), 1 oz. 15
ham, see "Chicken ham"
roll, sliced (*Longacre*), 1 oz. 25
white meat, oven-roasted (*Louis Rich*), 1 oz. 16

Chicken dinner, frozen:
à la king (*Armour Classics Lite*), 11.25 oz. 55
breast marsala (*Armour Classics Lite*), 10.5 oz. . . . 80
burgundy (*Armour Classics Lite*), 10 oz. 45
cacciatore (*The Budget Gourmet*), 11 oz. 60
and dumplings (*Banquet*), 10 oz. 45
fettuccine (*Armour Classics*), 11 oz. 50
glazed (*Armour Classics*), 10.75 oz. 60
glazed, breast (*Le Menu* LightStyle), 10 oz. 55
herb roasted (*Healthy Choice*), 11 oz. 40
herb roasted (*Le Menu* LightStyle), 10 oz. 70
mesquite (*Armour Classics*), 9.5 oz. 55
mesquite (*Healthy Choice*), 10.5 oz. 45
Mexicana (*The Budget Gourmet*), 12.8 oz. 40
and noodles (*Armour Classics*), 11 oz. 50
nuggets (*Kid Cuisine*), 6.25 oz. 60
Oriental (*Armour Classics Lite*), 10 oz. 35
Oriental (*Healthy Choice*), 11.25 oz. 55
parmigiana (*Armour Classics*), 11.5 oz. 75
parmigiana (*Healthy Choice*), 11.5 oz. 60
and pasta divan (*Healthy Choice*), 11.5 oz. 60
roast (*The Budget Gourmet*), 11.2 oz. 40
sweet and sour (*Armour Classics Lite*), 11 oz. 35
sweet and sour (*Healthy Choice*), 11.5 oz. 50
teriyaki (*The Budget Gourmet*), 12 oz. 55

Chicken dinner *(cont.)*
  w/wine and mushroom sauce *(Armour Classics)*,
    10.75 oz. 50

Chicken entrée, canned or packaged:
  Acapulco *(Hormel Top Shelf)*, 1 serving 55
  breast of, glazed *(Hormel Top Shelf)*, 1 serving . . . 75
  chow mein *(La Choy Bi-Pack)*, 3/4 cup 18
  sweet and sour *(Hormel Top Shelf)*, 1 serving 60

Chicken entrée, frozen:
  à la king:
    (Dining Lite), 9 oz. 40
    (Le Menu LightStyle), 8.25 oz. 30
    (Weight Watchers), 9 oz. 20
  almond, w/rice and vegetables *(La Choy Fresh &*
    Light), 9.75 oz. 42
  à l'orange *(Healthy Choice)*, 9 oz. 45
  à l'orange, w/almond rice *(Lean Cuisine)*, 8 oz. . . . 55
  au gratin *(The Budget Gourmet)*, 9.1 oz. 70
  breast, boneless:
    chunks *(Tyson)*, 3 oz. 30
    fillets *(Tyson)*, 3 oz. 25
    in herb cream sauce *(Lean Cuisine)*, 9.5 oz. 80
    marsala, w/vegetables *(Lean Cuisine)*, 8 1/8 oz. . . 80
    Parmesan *(Lean Cuisine)*, 10 oz. 80
  breast tenders, Southern fried *(Tyson)*, 3 oz. 25
  cacciatore *(Lean Cuisine)*, 10 7/8 oz. 45
  w/cheddar *(Tyson Chick'n Cheddar)*, 2.6 oz. 40
  chow mein:
    (Dining Lite), 9 oz. 30
    (Healthy Choice), 8.5 oz. 45
    w/rice *(Lean Cuisine)*, 11.25 oz. 35
  chunks *(Tyson Chick'n Chunks)*, 2.6 oz. 35
  chunks, Southern fried *(Tyson Chick'n Chunks)*,
    2.6 oz. 35
  cordon bleu *(Weight Watchers)*, 8 oz. 50
  diced *(Tyson)*, 3 oz. 70

Dijon *(Le Menu* LightStyle), 8 oz. 40
and egg noodles, w/broccoli *(The Budget
 Gourmet),* 10 oz. 130
empress *(Le Menu* LightStyle), 8.25 oz. 30
enchilada, see "Enchilada entrée"
fajita, see "Fajita entrée"
w/fettuccine *(The Budget Gourmet),* 10 oz. 100
fiesta *(Healthy Choice),* 8.5 oz. 45
French recipe *(The Budget Gourmet* Slim Selects),
 10 oz. 60
fried, Southern *(Weight Watchers),* 6.5 oz. 65
fried, white meat, regular or hot'n spicy *(Banquet
 Platter),* 9 oz. 105
glazed:
 (Dining Lite), 9 oz. 45
 (Healthy Choice), 8.5 oz. 50
 w/vegetable rice *(Lean Cuisine),* 8.5 oz. 55
herb roasted *(Le Menu* LightStyle), 7.75 oz. 45
imperial *(Weight Watchers),* 9.25 oz. 35
imperial, w/rice *(La Choy Fresh & Lite),* 11 oz. . . . 46
Italiano, w/fettuccine and vegetables *(Right
 Course),* 9⅝ oz. 45
Kiev *(Weight Watchers),* 7 oz. 30
mandarin *(The Budget Gourmet),* 10 oz. 25
and noodles *(Dining Lite),* 9 oz. 50
and noodles, homestyle *(Weight Watchers),* 9 oz. 30
nuggets *(Weight Watchers),* 5.9 oz. 50
Oriental *(Lean Cuisine),* 9⅜ oz. 100
Oriental, spicy *(La Choy Fresh & Lite),* 9.75 oz. . . . 42
patties:
 (Tyson), 2.6 oz. 35
 (Tyson Thick & Crispy), 2.6 oz. 40
 breast, Southern fried *(Tyson),* 2.6 oz. 35
pie:
 (Banquet), 7 oz. 35
 (Banquet Supreme Microwave), 7 oz. 40
 (Morton), 7 oz. 35
sandwich, see "Chicken sandwich"

Chicken entrée, frozen *(cont.)*
sesame *(Right Course)*, 10 oz. 50
sweet and sour:
   w/rice *(The Budget Gourmet)*, 10 oz. 40
   w/rice and vegetables *(La Choy Fresh & Lite)*,
     10 oz. 53
   tenders *(Weight Watchers)*, 10.19 oz. 40
tenderloins, in barbecue sauce *(Right Course)*,
   8.75 oz. 40
tenderloins, in peanut sauce *(Right Course)*,
   9.25 oz. 50
w/vegetables and vermicelli *(Lean Cuisine)*,
   11.75 oz. 45

Chicken entrée, refrigerated, 5 oz.:
bleu cheese, cajun, or mustard and dill *(Chicken By
   George)* 80
lemon herb *(Chicken By George)* 70
mesquite barbecue *(Chicken By George)* 70
teriyaki *(Chicken By George)* 65
tomato herb and basil *(Chicken By George)* 90

Chicken fat:
1 oz. 16

Chicken frankfurter:
(Longacre), 1 oz. 30
batter-wrapped *(Tyson Corn Dogs)*, 3.5 oz. 75

Chicken giblets, broiled-fryer, simmered:
4 oz. 446
chopped, 1 cup 570

Chicken gravy:
canned *(Heinz)*, 2 oz. 1

Chicken ham:
(Pilgrim's Pride), 1-oz. slice 18

The Cholesterol Content of Food

Chicken liver, see "Liver"

Chicken luncheon meat, see "Chicken, luncheon
meat and boneless"

Chicken salad:
    (Longacre/Longacre Saladfest), 1 oz.   15

Chicken sandwich, frozen:
    (MicroMagic), 4.5 oz.   35

Chicken seasoning and coating mix:
    (Golden Dipt)   0
    (McCormick/Schilling Bag'n Season)   0
    all varieties *(Shake'n Bake)*   0
    all varieties *(Shake'n Bake Oven Fry)*   0

Chicken side dish mix*:
    meatless style *(Hain)*   0

Chicken spread:
    chunky *(Underwood* Light), 2 1/8 oz.   30
    chunky or smokey flavor *(Underwood),* 2 1/8 oz. . . .   40

Chick-peas:
    dry or canned, plain (all brands)   0

Chicory, witloof:
    fresh   0

Chicory greens:
    fresh   0

Chicory root:
    1 medium   0

Chili, canned:
    (Old El Paso Chili Con Carne), 1 cup   47
    w/beans *(Hormel Micro-Cup),* 7.5 oz.   65

Chili *(cont.)*
w/beans *(Old El paso)*, 1 cup 32
w/beans, hot *(Gebhardt)*, 4 oz. 17
w/chicken, spicy *(Hain)*, 7.5 oz. 40
tempeh, spicy *(Hain)*, 7.5 oz. 0
vegetarian (all brands) 0

Chili beans, canned:
(Hunt's) 0
spiced *(Gebhardt)* 0

Chili entree, frozen:
vegetarian *(Right Course)*, 9.75 oz. 0

Chili entree, packaged:
con carne suprema *(Hormel Top Shelf)*, 1 serving 65

Chili mix:
(Gebhardt Chili Quik) 0

Chili pepper, see "Pepper, chili"

Chili powder:
all blends (all brands) 0

Chili sauce:
(Del Monte) 0
(Heinz) 0
(S&W Chili Makin's) 0
green, mild *(El Molino)* 0

Chili seasoning mix:
(Lawry's Seasoning Blends) 0
(McCormick/Schilling) 0
mild or hot *(Hain)* 0

Chimichanga entree, frozen:
bean and cheese *(Old El Paso)*, 1 piece 20

Chitterlings, pork:
simmered, 4 oz. 162

Chives:
fresh or freeze-dried 0

Chocolate, see "Candy"

Chocolate, baking:
bars, unsweetened *(Hershey's)*, 1 oz. 0
chips:
  milk *(Baker's)*, 1 oz. 5
  milk *(Baker's* Big Chip), 1/4 cup 10
  milk *(Hershey's)*, 1 oz. 10
  all varieties, except milk *(Hershey's)*, 1/4 cup . . . 0
shreds *(Tone's)*, 1 tsp. 0

Chocolate flavor drink:
canned, all varieties *(Sego/Sego* Lite), 10 oz. 5
mix *(Hershey's)* 0
mix *(Nestlé Quik)* 0
mix *(Pillsbury* Instant Breakfast) 0

Chocolate milk:
8 fl. oz. 30
lowfat 2% *(Darigold)*, 8 fl. oz. 17
lowfat 2% *(Hershey's)*, 8 fl. oz. 20

Chocolate mousse:
frozen *(Weight Watchers)*, 2.5 oz. 5
mix, w/whole milk, all varieties *(Jell-O Rich &*
Luscious), 1/2 cup 10

Chocolate syrup:
(Hershey's) 0
(Nestlé Quik) 0
flavored *(Smucker's)* 0

Chocolate topping:
fudge *(Hershey's)*, 2 tbsp. 5
regular or hot fudge *(Kraft)*, 1 tbsp. 0

Chow mein, see specific dinner and entree listings

Chow mein noodles, see "Noodle, Chinese"

Chrysanthemum garland:
raw or boiled 0

Chub, see "Cisco"

Cinnamon:
ground or stick 0

Cisco, meat only:
smoked, 4 oz. 36

Citrus fruit drink, juice, or punch:
all varieties (all brands) 0

Citrus salad:
(Florigold) 0

Clam, meat only:
raw, 1 oz. 10
raw, 9 large or 20 small, 6.3 oz. 60
boiled, poached, or steamed, 4 oz. 76
canned, minced *(Progresso)*, 1/2 cup 31
frozen, fried *(Mrs. Paul's)*, 2.5 oz. 15
frozen, strips, crunchy *(Gorton's* Microwave
Specialty), 3.5 oz. 30

Clam dip:
(Breakstone's/Sealtest), 2 tbsp. 15
(Breakstone's Gourmet Chesapeake), 2 tbsp. 20
(Kraft), 2 tbsp. 10
(Kraft Premium), 2 tbsp. 20

Clam sauce:
canned, red or white *(Ferrara)*, 4 oz. 10

canned, white *(Progresso* Authentic Pasta Sauces),
  1/2 cup 19
refrigerated, red *(Contadina Fresh),* 7.5 oz. 35
refrigerated, white *(Contadina Fresh),* 6 oz. 94

Cloves, whole or ground:
  (all brands) 0

Coating mix, see specific listings

Cocktail sauce:
  all varieties (all brands) 0

Cocoa:
  powder *(Bensdorp),* 1 oz. . . . . <1
  powder, plain or European *(Hershey's)* 0
  mix, dry:
    (Carnation 70 Calorie), 1 pkt. 1
    chocolate, double rich *(Swiss Miss),* 1 pkt. 0
    chocolate, milk *(Swiss Miss),* 1 pkt. . . . . <1
    fudge *(Carnation),* 1 pkt. 1
    w/mini marshmallows *(Swiss Miss),* 1 oz. 0

Coconut:
  fresh, canned, dried, or packaged 0

Coconut cream:
  canned, sweetened (all brands) 0

Coconut milk or water:
  fresh or canned 0

Cod, meat only:
  fresh:
    Atlantic, raw, 1 lb. 195
    Atlantic, raw, 1 oz. 12
    Atlantic, baked, broiled, or microwaved, 4 oz. . . 62
    Pacific, raw, 1 lb. 168

Cod, fresh *(cont.)*
Pacific, raw, 1 oz.   10
canned, Atlantic, w/liquid, 4 oz.   62
dried, Atlantic, salted, 1 oz.   42
frozen *(Van de Kamp's* Natural), 4 oz.   25

Cod entrée, frozen:
(Mrs. Paul's Light Fillets), 1 piece   50
(Van de Kamp's Light), 1 piece   35
oven fried *(Weight Watchers),* 7.08 oz.   15

Cod liver oil, see "Oil"

Coffee:
plain, ground, instant, or freeze-dried   0
flavored, all varieties *(General Foods* International)   0

Coffee, substitute, cereal grain beverage:
powder (all brands)   0

Coffee liqueur:
53 proof   0

Cold cuts, see specific listings

Collards:
fresh, canned, or frozen, plain   0

Cookies, 1 piece, except as noted:
animal crackers:
(Barnum's), 5 pieces   0
(FFV), 1.25-oz. pkg.   0
(Keebler), 5 pieces   0
(Sunshine), 13 pieces   0
apple bar *(Apple Newtons)*   0
apple n'raisin *(Archway)*   10
apricot-raspberry *(Pepperidge Farm* Fruit Cookies),
2 pieces   10
apricot-raspberry *(Pepperidge Farm* Zurich)   0

arrowroot biscuit *(National)* . . . . <2
assorted *(Archway* Select) 5
brownie:
   chocolate nut *(Pepperidge Farm* Old Fashioned)   5
   cream sandwich *(Pepperidge Farm* Capri) 0
   nut *(Pepperidge Farm* Beacon Hill) 5
butter flavor:
   (Pepperidge Farm Chessmen), 2 pieces 10
   chocolate coated *(Keebler* Baby Bear), 3 pieces   0
   chocolate coated *(Keebler E.L. Fudge),* 2 pieces   <5
chocolate, see "chocolate fudge," below
chocolate chip or chunk:
   (Almost Home Real) . . . . <2
   (Archway) 5
   (Chips Ahoy! Pure) 0
   (Drake's), 2 pieces 0
   (Grandma's Big Cookies), 2 pieces 5
   (Keebler Deluxe) . . . . <5
   (Pepperidge Farm Old Fashioned), 2 pieces . . . 5
   all varieties *(Keebler* Soft Batch) 0
   w/candy-coated chocolate *(Keebler Rainbow*
     Deluxe) . . . . <5
   chewy *(Chips Ahoy!)* . . . . <2
   chocolate *(Drake's),* 2 pieces 0
   chocolate, chunk *(Chips Ahoy!* Selections) 10
   chocolate, w/chocolate *(Keebler Magic Middles)*   <5
   chocolate walnut *(Chips Ahoy!* Selections) 5
   chunk *(Pepperidge Farm* Nantucket) 5
   chunk, pecan *(Chips Ahoy!* Selections) 10
   chunk, pecan *(Pepperidge Farm* Chesapeake) . . 5
   chunk, pecan *(Pepperidge Farm* Special
     Collection) 10
   chunky *(Chips Ahoy!* Selections) 10
   fudge *(Almost Home)* . . . . <2
   fudge *(Grandma's* Big Cookies), 2 pieces 5
   milk, macadamia *(Pepperidge Farm* Sausalito) . . 5
   milk, macadamia *(Pepperidge Farm* Special
     Collection) . . . . <5

Cookies, chocolate chip or chunk *(cont.)*

mini *(Mini Chips Ahoy!)*, 6 pieces or 1/2 oz.	0
snaps *(Nabisco)*, 3 pieces or 1/2 oz.	<2
sprinkled *(Chips Ahoy!)*	0
striped *(Chips Ahoy!)*	0
chocolate fudge:	
middles *(Nabisco)*	<5
mint *(Keebler Grasshopper)*, 2 pieces	0
snaps *(Nabisco)*, 4 pieces or 1/2 oz.	0
wafer *(Nabisco Famous Wafers)*, 1/2 oz.	<2
chocolate sandwich:	
(Little Debbie)	<1
(Oreo)	<2
(Oreo Big Stuf)	<5
(Oreo Double Stuf)	<2
fudge or white fudge covered *(Oreo)*	<2
fudge creme filled *(Keebler* Chocolate Creme Sandwich)	0
fudge, fudge creme filled *(Keebler E.L. Fudge)*	0
fudge, peanut butter creme filled *(Keebler E.L. Fudge)*	0
chocolate-filled sandwich:	
(Pepperidge Farm Brussels), 2 pieces	0
(Pepperidge Farm Lido)	<5
(Pepperidge Farm Milano), 2 pieces	5
fudge creme *(Keebler E.L. Fudge)*	<5
mint *(Pepperidge Farm* Brussels Mint), 2 pieces	0
mint or orange *(Pepperidge Farm* Milano), 2 pieces	5
chocolate peanut bar *(Ideal)*	0
coconut *(Drake's)*, 2 pieces	0
coconut, chocolate filled *(Pepperidge Farm* Tahiti)	5
coffee, chocolate-praline filled *(Pepperidge Farm* Cappuccino)	<5
creme sandwich, see specific listings	
date pecan *(Pepperidge Farm* Kitchen Hearth)	5
devil's food cake *(Nabisco)*	0

fig bar:
(Fig Newtons) 0
(Keebler) 0
vanilla *(FFV)* 0
whole wheat *(FFV)* 0
fudge bar, caramel and peanut *(Heyday)* 0
ginger *(Pepperidge Farm* Gingerman), 2 pieces . . . 5
ginger *(FFV)*, 1.25-oz. pkg. 0
gingersnap:
(Archway) 0
(FFV), 5 pieces 0
(Nabisco Old Fashioned) 0
(Sunshine), 5 pieces 0
graham cracker:
(Nabisco), 2 pieces 0
(Sunshine Grahamy Bears), 9 pieces 0
all varieties *(Honey Maid/Honey Maid* Graham
Bites) 0
all varieties *(Keebler)* 0
all varieties *(Teddy Grahams/Bearwich's)* 0
cinnamon or honey *(Sunshine)*, 1 piece 0
graham cracker, chocolate:
(Nabisco) 0
(Nabisco Teddy Grahams), 11 pieces 0
w/fudge *(Nabisco Cookies'N Fudge)*, 1/2 oz. . . . 0
hazelnut *(Pepperidge Farm* Old Fashioned),
2 pieces 0
jelly tart *(FFV)* 0
lemon nut crunch *(Pepperidge Farm* Old
Fashioned), 2 pieces . . . . <5
marshmallow cake:
(Mallomars) 0
(Nabisco Puffs/Twirls) 0
(Pinwheels) 0
mint sandwich *(Mystic Mint)* . . . . <2
molasses:
(Archway) 10
(Grandma's Old Time Big Cookies), 2 pieces . . . 5

Cookies, molasses *(cont.)*
   (Nabisco Pantry) 0
   crisps *(Pepperidge Farm* Old Fashioned),
     2 pieces 0
  oat bran raisin *(Awrey's)* 0
  oatmeal:
   (Archway) 5
   (Archway Ruth's Golden) 5
   (Baker's Bonus) 0
   (Drake's), 2 pieces 0
   (FFV), 5 pieces 0
   (Keebler Old Fashion) 0
   (Little Debbie), 2.75 oz. . . . . <2
   (Sunshine), 2 pieces 0
   apple-filled *(Archway)* 5
   apple spice *(Grandma's* Big Cookies), 2 pieces 10
   chocolate *(Pepperidge Farm* Dakota) 5
   w/chocolate *(Keebler Magic Middles)* 0
   chocolate chunk *(Chips Ahoy!)* . . . . <5
   date-filled *(Archway)* 5
   iced *(Archway)* 5
   Irish *(Pepperidge Farm* Old Fashioned), 2 pieces 5
  oatmeal raisin:
   (Almost Home) . . . . <2
   (Archway) 5
   (Entenmann's), 2 pieces 0
   (Keebler Soft Batch) 0
   (Pepperidge Farm Old Fashioned), 2 pieces . . . 10
   (Pepperidge Farm Santa Fe) . . . . <5
   bran *(Archway)* 5
  peach-apricot bar, vanilla *(FFV)* 0
  peach-apricot bar, whole wheat *(FFV)* 0
  peanut, chocolate-filled *(Pepperidge Farm* Nassau) <5
  peanut butter:
   (Grandma's Big Cookies), 2 pieces 10
   chocolate chip *(Keebler Soft Batch)* 0
   cream-filled *(Pitter Patter)* 0
   nut *(Keebler Soft Batch)* 0

sandwich *(Nutter Butter)* . . . . <2
peanut creme patties *(Nutter Butter)*, 2 pieces . . . 0
pecan crunch *(Archway)* 5
praline pecan *(FFV)* . . . . <5
raisin:
  bar, iced *(Keebler)* 0
  bran *(Pepperidge Farm* Kitchen Hearth) 0
  oatmeal *(Archway)* 0
  soft *(Grandma's* Big Cookies), 2 pieces 10
raspberry filled:
  (Pepperidge Farm Chantilly) . . . . <5
  (Pepperidge Farm Linzer) . . . . <5
  (Raspberry Newtons) 0
shortbread:
  (Lorna Doone), 3 pieces or 1/2 oz. . . . . <5
  (Pepperidge Farm Old Fashioned), 2 pieces . . . <5
  w/chocolate cream center *(Keebler Magic*
    Middles) . . . . <5
  country *(FFV)* . . . . <5
  fudge-striped *(Keebler* Fudge Stripes) 0
  fudge-striped *(Nabisco Cookies 'N Fudge)* 0
  pecan *(Nabisco)* . . . . <2
  pecan *(Pecan Sandies)* . . . . <5
  pecan *(Pepperidge Farm* Old Fashioned) 0
(Social Tea) . . . . <2
strawberry *(Pepperidge Farm* Fruit Cookies),
  2 pieces 10
strawberry bar *(Strawberry Newtons)* 0
sugar *(Almost Home* Old Fashioned) . . . . <2
sugar *(Pepperidge Farm* Old Fashioned), 2 pieces 10
sugar wafer *(Biscos)*, 4 pieces 0
vanilla:
  (Pepperidge Farm Bordeaux), 2 pieces 0
  (Pepperidge Farm Pirouettes), 2 pieces . . . . . . <5
  chocolate laced *(Pepperidge Farm* Pirouettes),
    2 pieces . . . . <5
  chocolate nut-coated *(Pepperidge Farm* Geneva),
    2 pieces 0

Cookies, vanilla *(cont.)*
creme sandwich *(Cameo)* 0
creme sandwich *(Keebler* French Vanilla Creme) 0
creme sandwich *(Nabisco Cookie Break)* 0
creme sandwich *(Nabisco Giggles)* . . . . <2
wafer *(Archway)* 0
wafer *(FFV),* 1 oz. . . . . <5
wafer *(Nilla* Wafers), 1/2 oz. . . . . <5
wafer, cinnamon *(Nilla* Wafers), 1/2 oz. . . . . <5
wafer, golden *(Keebler),* 4 pieces 0
wafer (see also specific listings):
brown edged *(Nabisco),* 1/2 oz. . . . . <2
creme, fudge covered *(Keebler Fudge Sticks),*
2 pieces 0
fudge *(Nabisco Cookies'N Fudge)* 0
waffle cremes *(Biscos),* 2 pieces or 1/2 oz. 0

Cookies, refrigerated:
all varieties, except oatmeal raisin *(Pillsbury),*
1 piece 5
oatmeal raisin *(Pillsbury),* 1 piece 0

Coriander:
fresh or dried 0

Corn:
fresh, canned, or frozen, w/out sauce 0
canned, w/beans, carrots, pasta, tomato sauce
(Green Giant Pantry Express), 1/2 cup 0
frozen, in butter sauce:
(The Budget Gourmet Side Dish), 5.5 oz. 15
(Green Giant Niblets One Serving), 4.5 oz. 5
(Stokely Singles), 4 oz. 5
on cob *(Stokely Singles),* 1 ear 5
golden or white *(Green Giant),* 1/2 cup 5
tender, sweet *(Birds Eye* Combination), 3.3 oz. . . . 5
frozen, country style *(The Budget Gourmet* Side
Dish), 5.75 oz. 15
frozen, nuggets *(Stilwell Quickkrisp),* 3 oz. 1

The Cholesterol Content of Food

Corn bran:
crude   0

Corn cake:
(Quaker Grain Cakes)   0

Corn chips and similar snacks, 1 oz.:
(Dipsy Doodles Rippled)   0
(Planters) . . . .
(Snyder's)   0
(Wise Corn Chips/Crunchies/*Ridgies)*   0
all varieties *(Bachman)*   0
all varieties *(Fritos/Fritos Crisp'N Thin)*   0
cheese *(Chee·tos* Balls, Crunchy, or Puffs) . . . . .   tr.
cheese *(Planters* Balls or Curls)   5
tortilla:
  (La Famous)   0
  (Old El Paso/Old El Paso Nachips)   0
  all varieties *(Bearitos)*   0
  all varieties *(Doritos)*   0
  all varieties *(Tostitos)*   0
  nacho, strips, or jalapeño flavor *(Bravos)*   0
  ranch *(Eagle)*   1
  sesame *(Hain)*   0
  sesame, cheese, or taco style *(Hain)* . . . .   <5

Corn flake crumbs:
(Kellogg's)   0

Corn flour:
all varieties   0

Corn fritter, frozen:
(Mrs. Paul's), 2 pieces   10

Corn grits:
plain, dry, all varieties   0
instant, w/imitation bacon or ham bits *(Quaker)* . . .   0

Corn oil, see "Oil"

Corn syrup:
dark or light *(Karo)* 0

Cornbread mix:
(Aunt Jemima Easy), 1 serving* 13
(Martha White Cotton Pickin'), 1/4 pan* 2
yellow *(Martha White* Light Crust), 2 oz. 26

Cornish game hen:
frozen *(Tyson),* 3.5 oz. 75

Cornmeal:
white or yellow, plain (all brands) 0

Cornmeal mix:
buttermilk, white or yellow 0

Cornstarch:
(Argo/Kingsford) 0

Cottonseed kernels:
roasted 0

Cottonseed meal:
partially defatted 0

Country coating mix:
mild *(Shake'n Bake)* 0

Couscous:
dry or cooked, plain 0
pilaf mix, dry *(Casbah)* 0

Cowpeas:
fresh, canned, or frozen 0
fresh, leafy tips or pods 0

Cowpeas, catjang, see "Catjang"

Crab, meat only:
Alaska king:

raw, 1 lb.	189
raw, 1 oz.	12
boiled, poached, or steamed, 4 oz.	60

blue:

raw, 1 lb.	355
raw, 1 oz.	22
boiled, poached, or steamed, 4 oz.	113
canned, 4 oz.	101
Dungeness, raw, 1 oz.	17
queen, raw, 1 oz.	16

Crab, deviled, frozen:

(Mrs. Paul's), 1 piece	20
miniatures *(Mrs. Paul's),* 3.5 oz.	20

Crab, imitation (from surimi):

1 oz.	6
(Icicle Brand), 3.5 oz.	10

Crabapple:

fresh or canned	0

Crackers, 1/2 oz., except as noted:

all varieties *(Pepperidge Farm* Snack Sticks)	0
bacon flavor *(Keebler* Toasteds), 4 pieces	0
bacon flavor thins *(Nabisco)*	0
w/bacon and cheese *(Handi-Snacks),* 1 pkg.	20
bran, toasted *(Bran Thins),* 7 pieces	0

butter or butter flavor:

(Escort)	0
(Keebler Club Low Salt), 4 pieces	0
(Keebler Toasteds Buttercrisp), 4 pieces	0
(Keebler Town House), 4 pieces	0
(Pepperidge Farm Distinctive), 4 pieces	<5
(Ritz/Ritz Bits Regular/Low Salt)	0

Crackers, butter or butter flavor *(cont.)*
    dairy *(American Classic)*, 4 pieces . . . .   <2
  cheese:
    (Cheddar Wedges), 1/2 oz. or 31 pieces . . . . . .   <2
    (Cheese Nips) . . . .   <2
    (Cheez-It Regular/Low Salt), 12 pieces . . . .   <2
    (Ritz Bits) . . . .   <2
    (Tid Bits) . . . .   <2
    cheddar *(Better Cheddars)* . . . .   <2
    cheddar *(Keebler Town House Jrs.)*, 8 pieces . . .   <5
    cheddar *(Pepperidge Farm* Goldfish), 1 oz.   5
    Parmesan *(Pepperidge Farm* Tiny Goldfish), 1 oz.   <5
    Swiss *(Nabisco Swiss Cheese)* . . . .   <2
    thins *(Pepperidge Farm* Goldfish), 4 pieces   0
  cheese sandwich:
    American, and wheat *(Keebler)*, 1 piece . . . . . .   <5
    cheddar *(Keebler Town House* & Cheddar),
      1 piece . . . .   <5
    and cheese *(Handi-Snacks)*, 1 pkg.   20
    and peanut butter *(Keebler)*, 2 pieces   0
  (Chicken In A Biskit)   0
  crispbread (see also specific cracker listings):
    all varieties *(Finn Crisp)*   0
    all varieties *(Kavli)*   0
    all varieties *(Ryvita)*   0
    all varieties *(Wasa)*   0
  (FFV Schooners)   0
  graham, see "Cookies"
  grain, mixed *(Harvest Crisps* 5 Grain)   0
  (Hain Rich)   0
  matzo, 1 board:
    all varieties, except egg *(Manischewitz)*   0
    egg *(Manischewitz* Passover)   25
    egg n' onion *(Manischewitz)*   15
  melba toast:
    all varieties *(Devonsheer)*   0
    all varieties *(Old London)*   0
  oat *(Oat Thins)*   0

The Cholesterol Content of Food

oat bran *(Oat Bran Krisp)* 0
onion *(Hain)*, 1 oz. 0
onion *(Keebler* Toasteds), 4 pieces 0
onion, minced *(American Classic)*, 4 pieces 0
peanut butter:
   and cheese *(Handi-Snacks)*, 1 pkg. 0
   cheese or toasty *(Little Debbie)*, .93 oz. . . . . . . <1
   sandwich *(Ritz Bits)* 0
   toast and *(Keebler)*, 2 pieces 0
(Pepperidge Farm Original Goldfish), 1 oz. 0
pizza flavor *(Pepperidge Farm* Goldfish), 1 oz. . . . <5
poppy, toasted *(American Classic)*, 4 pieces 0
pretzel *(Pepperidge Farm* Goldfish), 1 oz. 0
rye:
   (Hain), 1 oz. 0
   (Keebler Toasteds), 4 pieces 0
   all varieties *(Rykrisp)* 0
saltine:
   (Sunshine Krispy Regular/Unsalted Tops),
     5 pieces 0
   all varieties *(Premium)* 0
   original or wheat *(Zesta)*, 5 pieces 0
sesame:
   (FFV Crisp), 1 piece 0
   (Keebler Toasteds), 4 pieces 0
   (Pepperidge Farm Distinctive), 4 pieces 0
   bread wafer *(Meal Mates)* 0
   golden *(American Classic)*, 4 pieces 0
   wafer *(FFV* Crisp), 4 pieces 0
sesame and cheese *(Twigs* Snack Sticks) . . . . . . <2
soda or water:
   (Crown Pilot) 0
   (FFV Ocean Crisps), 1 piece 0
   (Pepperidge Farm English Water Biscuit),
     4 pieces 0
   (Royal Lunch) . . . . <2
   (Sailor Boy Pilot), 1 piece 0
soup and oyster *(Dandy/Oysterettes)* 0

Crackers *(cont.)*
  soup and oyster *(Sunshine)*, 16 pieces   0
  sourdough *(Hain)*   0
  toast *(Uneeda* Biscuits Unsalted Tops)   0
  vegetable *(Hain)*, 1 oz.   0
  vegetable *(Vegetable Thins)*, 7 pieces   0
  (Waverly)   0
  wheat:
    (FFV Stoned Wheat Wafer), 4 pieces   0
    (Ryvita Original Snackbread), 1 piece   0
    (Sociables), 6 pieces   0
    (Sunshine Wheats), 8 pieces   0
    (Triscuit/Triscuit Bits)   0
    (Wheat Thins)   0
    (Wheatsworth Stone Ground)   0
    cracked *(American Classic)*   0
    cracked or hearty *(Pepperidge Farm* Distinctive)   0
    nutty *(Wheat Thins)*   0
    toasted *(Pepperidge Farm)*, 4 pieces   0
    whole *(Keebler Wheatables)*, 12 pieces   0
    whole grain *(Keebler Harvest Wheats)*, 4 pieces   0
    wheat'n bran *(Triscuit)*   0

Cracker crumbs, see "Matzo crumbs and meal"

Cranberry:
  fresh, canned, or frozen   0

Cranberry beans:
  cooked or canned   0

Cranberry drink or juice:
  all blends (all brands)   0

Cranberry fruit concentrate:
  (Hain)   0

The Cholesterol Content of Food

Cranberry-orange relish:
fresh or canned 0

Cranberry sauce:
whole or jellied, all blends (all brands) 0

Crayfish, meat only:
raw, 1 lb. 628
raw, 1 oz., 8 medium 39
boiled or steamed, 4 oz. 202

Cream:
half and half, 1 cup 89
half and half, 1 tbsp. 6
light, coffee or table, 1 cup 159
light, coffee or table, 1 tbsp. 10
medium (25% fat), 1 cup 209
medium (25% fat), 1 tbsp. 13
sour, see "Cream, sour" and "Cream, sour,
nondairy"
whipped topping:
(La Creme), 1 tbsp. . . . . <1
frozen (Kraft Real Cream), 1/4 cup 10
nondairy, see "Cream topping, nondairy"
pressurized, 1 tbsp. 2
pressurized (Crowley), 1 tbsp. 5
whipping:
light, 1 cup (2 cups whipped) 265
light, 1 tbsp. (2 tbsp. whipped) 17
heavy, 1 cup (2 cups whipped) 326
heavy, 1 tbsp. (2 tbsp. whipped) 21

Cream, sour:
1 cup. 102
1 tbsp. 5
(Breakstone's/Sealtest), 1 tbsp. 10
(Crowley Light), 1 oz. 5
(Knudsen Hampshire), 1 oz. 20
(Knudsen Light N' Lively), 1 oz. 10

Cream, sour *(cont.)*
half and half:
1 oz. 11
1 tbsp. 6
(Sealtest Light/Breakstone's Light Choice),
1 tbsp. 5
imitation *(Pet/Dairymate),* 1 tbsp. . . . . <1
lowfat *(Friendship Lite Delite),* 1 oz. 8

Cream, sour, nondairy:
all varieties 0
dressing *(Crowley)* 0

Cream puff, frozen:
Bavarian *(Rich's),* 1 piece 25

Cream of tartar:
(Tone's) 0

Cream topping, dairy, see "Cream"

Cream topping, nondairy:
frozen, mix, or pressurized (all brands) 0

Creamer, nondairy:
(Crowley), 1/2 oz. 5
(Rich's Coffee Rich/Farm Rich/Poly Rich) 0
liquid *(Coffee-mate)* 0
powder *(Cremora)* 0

Crème de menthe:
72 proof 0

Creole sauce:
Cajun *(Enrico's Light)* 0

Cress, garden:
raw or boiled 0

Cress, water, see "Watercress"

Croaker, Atlantic, meat only:
raw, 1 lb.	277
raw, 1 oz.	17

Croissant:
butter *(Awrey's)*, 2-oz. piece	30
margarine or wheat *(Awrey's)*, 1 piece	5

Crookneck squash:
fresh, canned, or frozen, plain	0

Crouton, 1/2 oz.:
all varieties *(Pepperidge Farm)*	0
Caesar salad or seasoned *(Brownberry)*	<1
cheddar *(Brownberry)*	3
onion and garlic *(Brownberry)*	1
toasted *(Brownberry)*	0

Crowder peas, see "Peas, crowder"

Cucumber:
fresh	0

Cucumber dip:
creamy *(Kraft* Premium), 2 tbsp.	10

Cucumber and onion dip:
(Breakstone's/Sealtest), 2 tbsp.	15

Cumin:
seed or ground (all brands)	0

Cupcake, see "Cake, snack"

Currant:
all varieties, fresh or dried	0

Curry powder:
all blends (all brands) 0

Curry sauce mix:
1.25-oz. pkt. . . . . tr.

Cusk, meat only:
raw, 1 lb. 186
raw, 1 oz. 12

Custard, see "Pudding mix"

Custard apple:
fresh 0

Cuttlefish, meat only:
raw, 1 lb. 507
raw, 1 oz. 32

D

Food and Measure	Cholesterol (mgs.)
Daikon, see "Radish"	
Daiquiri mix:	
bottled or instant, all flavors *(Holland House)*	0
Dairy Queen/Brazier, 1 serving:	
sandwiches:	
BBQ beef, 4.5 oz.	20
chicken fillet, breaded, 6.7 oz.	55
chicken fillet, breaded, w/cheese, 7.2 oz.	70
chicken fillet, grilled, 6.5 oz.	50
fish fillet, 6 oz.	45
fish fillet, w/cheese, 6.5 oz.	60

Dairy Queen/Brazier, sandwiches *(cont.)*

hamburger:

single, 5 oz.	45
single, w/cheese, 5.5 oz.	60
double, 7 oz.	95
double, w/cheese, 8 oz.	120
DQ Homestyle Ultimate Burger, 9.7 oz.	140

hot dog:

3.5 oz.	25
w/cheese, 4 oz.	35
w/chili, 4.5 oz.	30
1/4 lb. *Super Dog,* 7 oz.	60

side dishes and dressings:

dressing, french, reduced calorie, 2 oz.	0
dressing, Thousand Island, 2 oz.	25
french fries	0
onion rings	0
salad, garden, w/out dressing, 10 oz.	185
salad, side, w/out dressing, 4.8 oz.	0

desserts and shakes:

banana split, 13 oz.	30

Blizzard:

Heath, small, 10.3 oz.	40
Heath, regular, 14.3 oz.	60
strawberry, small, 9.4 oz.	35
strawberry, regular, 13.5 oz.	50

Breeze:

Heath, small, 9.6 oz.	10
Heath, regular, 13.4 oz.	15
strawberry, small or regular	5
Brownie Delight, hot fudge, 10.8 oz.	35
Buster Bar, 5.3 oz.	15

cone:

chocolate or vanilla, regular, 5 oz.	20
chocolate or vanilla, large, 7.5 oz.	30
chocolate dipped, regular, 5.5 oz.	20
vanilla, small, 3 oz.	15
Dilly Bar, 3 oz.	10

The Cholesterol Content of Food

DQ frozen cake slice, undecorated, 5.8 oz.	20
DQ Sandwich, 2.2 oz.	5
malt, vanilla, regular, 14.7 oz.	45
Mr. Misty, regular, 11.6 oz.	0
Nutty Double Fudge, 9.7 oz.	35
Peanut Buster parfait, 10.8 oz.	30
QC Big Scoop, chocolate or vanilla, 4.5 oz.	35
shake, chocolate or vanilla, regular, 14 oz.	45
shake, vanilla, large, 16.3 oz.	50
sundae, chocolate, regular, 6.2 oz.	20
Waffle Cone Sundae, strawberry, 6.1 oz.	20
yogurt, cone or cup, regular or large	<5
yogurt, strawberry sundae, regular, 12.5 oz.	<5

Dandelion greens:

raw or cooked	0

Danish, 1 piece:

apple, fried *(Hostess Breakfast Bake Shop)*	20
cheese *(Awrey's* Round), 2.75 oz.	10
cinnamon raisin *(Awrey's* Square), 3 oz.	15
cinnamon walnut *(Awrey's* Round), 2.75 oz.	5
pineapple, miniature *(Awrey's),* 1.7 oz.	5
raspberry *(Awrey's* Square), 3 oz.	10
raspberry, fried *(Hostess Breakfast Bake Shop)*	20
strawberry *(Awrey's* Round), 2.75 oz.	5
refrigerated:	
caramel, w/nuts *(Pillsbury)*	0
cinnamon raisin *(Pillsbury)*	0
orange *(Pillsbury)*	0

Dasheen, see "Taro"

Date:

all varieties (all brands)	0

Diable sauce:

(Escoffier)	0

Dill dip:
creamy *(Nasoya Vegi-Dip)* 0

Dill seasoning:
(McCormick/Schilling Parsley Patch It's a Dilly) . . . 0

Dill seed or weed:
(all brands) 0

Dips, see specific listings

Dock:
raw or cooked 0

Dolphin fish, meat only:
raw, 1 lb. 331
raw, 1 oz. 21

Domino's Pizza, 2 slices:
cheese 19
deluxe 40
double cheese/pepperoni 48
ham 26
pepperoni 28
sausage/mushroom 28
veggie 36

Donut, 1 piece:
(Hostess Old Fashioned) 10
cinnamon *(Hostess Breakfast Bake Shop* Pantry) . . 10
cinnamon or cinnamon, apple filled *(Hostess
Breakfast Bake Shop Donette Gems)* 5
crumb *(Hostess Breakfast Bake Shop)*, 1¹/5 oz. . . 5
crumb *(Hostess Breakfast Bake Shop Donette
Gems)* 5
frosted *(Hostess Breakfast Bake Shop)*, 1.5 oz. . . . 5
frosted, plain, or strawberry filled *(Hostess
Breakfast Bake Shop Donette Gems)* . . . . <5
glazed *(Hostess* Old Fashioned) 15

glazed whirl *(Hostess Breakfast Bake Shop)* 5
honey wheat *(Hostess Breakfast Bake Shop)* 25
plain or frosted *(Hostess O's)* 5
plain or powdered sugar, assorted *(Hostess
   Breakfast Bake Shop Pantry)* 10
plain or powdered sugar *(Hostess Breakfast Bake
   Shop Donette Gems)* 5
powdered sugar, strawberry filled *(Hostess
   Breakfast Bake Shop Donette Gems)* 5
stick *(Little Debbie)* . . . . <1

Drum, freshwater, meat only:
raw, 1 lb. 290
raw, 1 oz. 18
Druther's, [1] *1 serving:*
breakfast:
   bacon and egg biscuit 253
   bacon and fried egg plate 500
   bacon and scrambled egg plate 501
   ham and egg biscuit 256
   ham and fried egg plate 511
   ham and scrambled egg plate 515
   sausage and egg biscuit 257
   sausage and fried egg plate 515
   sausage and scrambled egg plate 515
   1 sausage, 1 biscuit 17
biscuits and gravy 3
cheeseburger:
   regular 69
   deluxe quarter 127
   double 105
chicken:
   12-piece, 3.9 lbs. 902
   8-piece, 2.6 lbs. 601
   3-piece, breast, thigh, and leg, 1.1 lb. 273

[1] *Values for dishes and dinners are complete as served, including biscuits, potatoes, coleslaw, and hushpuppies.*

Druther's, chicken *(cont.)*
   breast and wing, 7.5 oz.   154
   breast and wing, w/potatoes and coleslaw,
      14 oz.   159
   thigh and drumstick, 6.9 oz.   152
   thigh and drumstick, w/potatoes and coleslaw,
      13.4 oz.   157
   Fish and Chips   112
   fish dinner   117
   fish sandwich   56
   hamburger   55

Duck, domesticated, roasted:
   meat w/skin, 4 oz.   95
   meat only, 4 oz.   101

Duck, wild, raw:
   meat w/skin, 1 oz.   23

Duck sauce, see "Sweet and sour sauce"

E

Food and Measure	Cholesterol (mgs.)
Eclair, chocolate, frozen:	
(Rich's), 1 piece	35
Eel, meat only:	
raw, 1 oz.	36
baked, broiled, or microwaved, 4 oz.	183
Egg, chicken:	
raw, fresh or frozen:	
whole, 1 large	213
white from 1 large egg	0
yolk from 1 large egg	213
cooked:	
hard-boiled, 1 large	213
hard-boiled, chopped, 1 cup	578

Egg, chicken, cooked *(cont.)*
poached, 1 large 212
dried, 1 oz.:
whole 544
whole, stabilized 572
white, stabilized, flakes 0
yolk 830

Egg, substitute or imitation:
(Fleischmann's Egg Beaters) 0
(Morningstar Farms Scramblers) 0
(Tofutti Egg Watchers) 0
w/cheez *(Fleischmann's Egg Beaters)*, 1/2 cup 5

Egg, duck, fresh:
whole, raw, 1 egg 619

Egg, quail, fresh:
whole, raw, 1 egg 76

Egg, turkey, fresh:
whole, raw, 1 egg 737

"Egg" breakfast, vegetarian, frozen:
Scramblers, hash browns and links *(Morningstar
Farms),* 7 oz. 0
Scramblers, pancakes and links *(Morningstar
Farms),* 6.8 oz. 0

Egg breakfast sandwich, frozen:
English muffin *(Weight Watchers),* 4 oz. 160

Egg roll, vegetarian, frozen:
(Worthington) 0

Egg roll wrapper:
(Nasoya) 0

Eggnog, nonalcoholic:
(*Crowley*), 6 fl. oz. 100

Eggplant:
raw or boiled, plain 0

Eggplant appetizer:
(*Progresso* Caponata) 0

Eggplant entrée, frozen:
parmigiana (*Mrs. Paul's*), 4 oz. 15

Elderberry:
fresh 0

Enchilada dinner, frozen:
beef (*Patio*), 13.25 oz. 40
cheese (*Patio*), 12.25 oz. 20

Enchilada entrée, frozen:
beef (*Old El Paso*), 1 piece 10
beef, sirloin Ranchero (*The Budget Gourmet*), 9 oz. . 35
beef Ranchero (*Weight Watchers*), 9.12 oz. 40
cheese Ranchero (*Weight Watchers*), 8.87 oz. 60
chicken:
   (*Le Menu* LightStyle), 8 oz. 35
   Suiza (*The Budget Gourmet*), 9 oz. 50
   Suiza (*Weight Watchers*), 9 oz. 30
vegetable, w/tofu (*Legume*), 11 oz. 0

Enchilada mix*:
(*Old El Paso* Dinner), 1 piece 21

Enchilada sauce:
(*Rosarita*) 0
all varieties (*Del Monte*) 0
all varieties (*Old El Paso*) 0
all varieties (*Ortega*) 0

Endive, curly:
   fresh 0

Endive, Belgian, see "Chicory, witloof"

Eppaw:
   fresh 0

Escarole, see "Endive"

F

Food and Measure	Cholesterol (mgs.)
Fajita entrée:	
frozen, beef *(Weight Watchers)*, 6.75 oz.	20
frozen, chicken *(Weight Watchers)*, 6.75 oz.	30
refrigerated, chicken *(Chicken By George)*, 5 oz. . .	85
Falafel mix:	
dry *(Casbah)*	0
Farina, whole-grain (see also "Cereal, cooking"):	
dry or cooked, plain	0
Fat, see specific listings	

Fat, imitation:
  (Rokeach Neutral Nyafat)   0

Fava beans, canned:
  (Progresso)   0

Fennel, fresh:
  (Frieda of California)   0

Fennel seed:
  (all brands)   0

Fenugreek seed:
  (all brands)   0

Fettucini entrée, frozen:
  Alfredo *(Healthy Choice)*, 8 oz.   45
  Alfredo *(Weight Watchers)*, 9 oz.   35
  w/broccoli *(Dining Lite)*, 9 oz.   35
  chicken *(Weight Watchers)*, 8.25 oz.   40
  w/meat sauce *(The Budget Gourmet)*, 10 oz.   25
  primavera *(Green Giant)*, 1 pkg.   25

Fig:
  all varieties, fresh, canned, or dried   0

Filbert:
  dried, dry-roasted, or oil-roasted   0

Finnan haddie, see "Haddock, smoked"

Fish, see specific listings

Fish batter mix, see "Fish seasoning and coating
  mix"

Fish cakes, frozen:
  (Mrs. Paul's), 2 pieces   20

Fish dinner, frozen (see also specific listings):

(Morton), 9.75 oz.	65
nuggets *(Kid Cuisine),* 7 oz.	45

Fish entrée, frozen (see also specific listings):

(Banquet Platters), 8.75 oz.	95
battered, 2 pieces, except as noted:	
(Gorton's Crispy)	35
(Gorton's Crunchy)	40
(Gorton's Crunchy Microwave)	30
(Gorton's Potato Crisp)	30
(Mrs. Paul's Batter Dipped)	60
(Mrs. Paul's Crunchy Batter)	22
(Van de Kamp's), 1 piece	20
portions *(Mrs. Paul's)*	33
breaded:	
(Gorton's Light Recipe), 1 piece	30
(Van de Kamp's), 2 pieces	35
(Van de Kamp's Large Crispy Microwave), 1 piece	
crispy *(Van de Kamp's* Microwave), 1 piece	15
portions *(Mrs. Paul's* Crispy Crunchy), 2 pieces	25
in butter sauce *(Mrs. Paul's* Light Fillets), 1 piece	40
Dijon *(Mrs. Paul's* Light), 8.75 oz.	60
fillet of:	
au gratin *(Weight Watchers),* 9.25 oz.	60
divan *(Lean Cuisine),* 12³/₈ oz.	85
Florentine *(Lean Cuisine),* 9 oz.	100
in herb sauce *(Gorton's),* 1 pkg.	90
jardiniere *(Lean Cuisine),* 11.25 oz.	110
fillets *(Mrs. Paul's* Crispy Crunchy), 2 pieces	22
Florentine *(Mrs. Paul's* Light), 8 oz.	95
Mornay *(Mrs. Paul's* Light), 9 oz.	80
sticks *(Mrs. Paul's* Crispy Crunchy), 4 pieces	25
sticks, battered, 4 pieces, except as noted:	
(Gorton's Crispy or Crunchy)	25
(Gorton's Crunchy Microwave), 6 pieces	35
(Gorton's Potato Crisp)	25

Fish entrée, sticks, battered *(cont.)*
   (Mrs. Paul's) 25
   (Van de Kamp's) 20
  sticks, breaded:
   (Mrs. Paul's Crispy Crunchy), 4 pieces 20
   (Van de Kamp's/Van de Kamp's Value Pack),
     4 pieces 20
   (Van de Kamp's Crispy Microwave), 3 pieces . . . 15
  tempura *(Gorton's Light Recipe)*, 1 piece 30

Fish seasoning and coating mix:
  (Shake'n Bake) 0
  all varieties *(Golden Dipt)* 0

Flatfish, meat only:
  raw, 1 lb. 217
  raw, 1 oz. 14
  baked, broiled, or microwaved, 4 oz. 77

Flavor enhancer:
  (Ac'cent) 0

Flounder:
  fresh, see "Flatfish"
  frozen *(Van de Kamp's* Natural), 4 oz. 35

Flounder entrée, frozen:
  (Mrs. Paul's Crunchy Batter), 2 pieces 40
  (Mrs. Paul's Light Fillets), 1 piece 50
  (Van de Kamp's Light), 1 piece 45
  stuffed *(Gorton's Microwave Entrees)*, 1 pkg. 120

Flour, see specific grain listings

Forestiera sauce:
  refrigerated *(Contadina Fresh)*, 7.5 oz. 15

Frankfurter, 1 link, except as noted:
  (Eckrich Lite) 25
  (Eckrich Lite Bunsize) 35

(JM) 16
(JM, 10/lb.) 22
(JM Jumbo), 2 oz. 27
(Oscar Mayer Light Wieners), 2-oz. link 30
(Oscar Mayer Wieners, 10/lb.), 1.6-oz. link 29
(Oscar Mayer Wieners, 8/lb.), 2-oz. link 36
(Oscar Mayer Bun Length) 27
(Oscar Mayer Bun Length Wieners, 8/lb.), 2-oz. link 34
bacon and cheddar (Oscar Mayer, 10/lb.) 29
beef:
   (Boar's Head), 1 oz. 15
   (Hebrew National) 15
   (JM) 20
   (JM, 10/lb.) 26
   (JM Jumbo) 33
   (Oscar Mayer, 8/lb.), 2-oz. link 35
   (Oscar Mayer, 10/lb.), 1.6-oz. link 28
   (Oscar Mayer Light), 2-oz. link 23
   (Oscar Mayer Bun Length, 8/lb.), 2-oz. link 34
   (Oscar Mayer Bun Length, 4/lb.), 4-oz. link 68
   w/cheddar (Oscar Mayer, 10/lb.), 1.6-oz. link . . . 27
cheese (JM German) 37
cheese (Oscar Mayer, 10/lb.), 1.6-oz. link 30
chicken, see "Chicken frankfurter"
cocktail (Oscar Mayer Little Wieners) 5
pork and beef (Boar's Head), 1 oz. 15
turkey, see "Turkey frankfurter"

"Frankfurter," vegetarian:
canned or frozen, all varieties (Worthington) 0

French toast, frozen:
(Aunt Jemima Original), 3 oz. 46
(Downflake), 2 slices 73
cinnamon swirl (Aunt Jemima), 3 oz. 41
w/cinnamon (Weight Watchers), 3 oz. 5

French toast breakfast, frozen:
w/links *(Weight Watchers)*, 4.5 oz. 15
vegetarian, cinnamon swirl, w/patty *(Morningstar
Farms)*, 6.5 oz. 0

Frosting, ready-to-use:
all flavors *(Betty Crocker Creamy Deluxe)* 0

Frozen dessert, see specific listings

Fructose:
(Featherweight) 0

Fruit, see specific listings

Fruit, mixed:
canned, dried, or frozen (all brands) 0

Fruit bar, frozen:
plain, all flavors (all brands) 0
w/cream, blueberry, peach, raspberry, or
strawberry *(Dole* Fruit & Cream)*, 1 bar 5

Fruit cocktail:
canned (all brands) 0

Fruit juice or juice drink:
all varieties (all brands) 0

Fruit and nut mix:
(Planter's Fruit 'n Nut) 0

Fruit punch:
all varieties (all brands) 0

Fruit salad:
all varieties (all brands) 0

Fruit snack:
    plain, roll or pouch, all varieties (all brands)   0

Fruit spread:
    all flavors (all brands)   0

Fruit syrup:
    all flavors (all brands)   0

Fudge, see "Candy"

Fudge topping, see "Chocolate topping"

G

Garlic salt:
(Lawry's) 0

Garlic spread:
concentrate (Lawry's) 0

Gelatin, unflavored:
(Knox) 0

Gelatin bar, frozen:
all flavors (Jell-O Gelatin Pops) 0

Gelatin dessert mix*:
all flavors (all brands) 0

Gelatin drink mix:
orange flavor (Knox) 0

Ginger, root:
fresh or dried 0
pickled, Japanese 0

Ginkgo nut:
raw, canned, or dried 0

Goat, meat only:
roasted, 4 oz. 85

Godfather's Pizza:
original cheese:
  mini, 1/4 pie 8
  small, 1/6 pie 15
  medium, 1/8 pie 15
  large, 1/10 pie 20
  large, hot slice, 1/8 pie 25
original combo:
  mini, 1/4 pie 10
  small, 1/6 pie 30

Godfather's Pizza, original combo *(cont.)*
medium, 1/8 pie	35
large, 1/10 pie	36
large, hot slice, 1/8 pie	45
thin crust cheese:	
small, 1/6 pie	10
medium, 1/8 pie	14
large, 1/10 pie	16
thin crust combo:	
small, 1/6 pie	25
medium, 1/8 pie	25
large, 1/10 pie	27
stuffed pie, cheese:	
small, 1/6 pie	25
medium, 1/8 pie	25
large, 1/10 pie	32
stuffed pie, combo:	
small, 1/6 pie	40
medium, 1/8 pie	43
large, 1/10 pie	48

Goose, domesticated, roasted:
meat w/skin, 4 oz.	103
meat only, 4 oz.	109

Goose fat:
1 oz.	28

Goose liver, see "Pâté"

Gooseberry:
fresh or canned	0

Gourd:
all varieties	0

Granola, see "Cereal, ready-to-eat"

The Cholesterol Content of Food

Granola and cereal bars, 1 piece:

all varieties *(Kellogg's Smart Start)* 0

all varieties *(Quaker Chewy)* . . . . <1

all varieties *(Sunbelt)* . . . . <1

caramel nut *(Quaker Granola Dipps)* 2

chocolate chip *(Quaker Granola Dipps)* 1

cocoa creme or peanut butter, chocolate coated

   (Hershey's) 5

peanut butter *(Quaker Granola Dipps)* 2

Grape:

fresh or canned, all varieties 0

Grape drink:

canned, bottled, chilled, or mix (all brands) 0

Grape juice:

all varieties (all brands) 0

Grapefruit:

fresh, canned, or chilled, all varieties 0

Grapefruit juice:

all varieties (all brands) 0

Gravy, see specific listings

Great northern beans:

raw, boiled, or canned, plain 0

Green beans:

fresh, canned, or frozen, w/out sauce 0

canned, w/potatoes and mushrooms, in sauce

   (Green Giant Pantry Express), 1/2 cup 0

frozen, in butter sauce *(Green Giant),* 1/2 cup 5

frozen, in butter sauce *(Green Giant* One Serving),

   5.5 oz. 5

Green beans, combinations, frozen:
Bavarian style, w/spaetzle *(Birds Eye)*, 3.3 oz. 10
French, w/toasted almonds *(Birds Eye*
Combinations), 3 oz. 0
and mushroom, creamy *(Green Giant* Garden
Gourmet), 1 pkg. 25

Grenadine:
(Rose's) 0

Grits, see "Corn grits"

Ground cherry:
fresh 0

Grouper, meat only:
raw, 1 lb. 166
raw, 1 oz. 10
baked, broiled, or microwaved, 4 oz. 53

Guacamole, see "Avocado dip"

Guacamole seasoning:
(Lawry's) 0

Guava:
all varieties 0

Guava fruit drink:
all blends (all brands) 0

Guava juice:
all varieties (all brands) 0

Guava sauce:
cooked 0

Guinea hen, raw:
meat only, 1 oz. 18

H

Food and Measure	Cholesterol (mgs.)
Haddock, meat only:	
fresh:	
raw, 1 lb.	261
raw, 1 oz.	16
baked, broiled, or microwaved, 4 oz.	84
smoked, 4 oz.	87
frozen *(Van de Kamp's* Natural), 4 oz.	20
Haddock entrée, frozen:	
(Mrs. Paul's Light Fillets), 1 piece	45
(Van de Kamp's Light), 1 piece	35
battered *(Mrs. Paul's* Crunchy Batter), 2 pieces	25
battered *(Van de Kamp's),* 2 pieces	30
breaded *(Van de Kamp's),* 2 pieces	25

Haddock entrée *(cont.)*
in lemon butter *(Gorton's Microwave Entrees),*
1 pkg. 100

Hake, see "Whiting"

Halibut, meat only:
raw, 1 lb. 146
raw, 1 oz. 9
baked, broiled, or microwaved, 4 oz. 46

Halibut entrée, frozen:
battered *(Van de Kamp's),* 2 pieces 10

Halvah, 1 bar:
(Fantastic Foods) 0

Ham, fresh, meat only, roasted:
whole leg:
lean w/fat, 4 oz. 105
lean w/fat, chopped or diced, 1 cup 131
lean only, 4 oz. 107
lean only, chopped or diced, 1 cup 131
rump half, lean w/fat, 4 oz. 108
rump half, lean only, 4 oz. 109
shank half, lean w/fat, 4 oz. 104
shank half, lean only, 4 oz. 104

Ham, canned:
(Oscar Mayer Jubilee), 1 oz. 14

Ham, cured (see also "Ham, canned"):
whole leg, lean w/fat:
unheated, 1 oz. 16
roasted, 4 oz. 70
roasted, chopped or diced, 1 cup 86
whole leg, lean only:
unheated, 1 oz. 15
roasted, 4 oz. 62

roasted, chopped or diced, 1 cup 78
boneless (11% fat):
  unheated, 1 oz. 16
  roasted, 4 oz. 67
  roasted, chopped or diced, 1 cup 83
boneless, extra lean (5% fat):
  unheated, 1 oz. 13
  roasted, 4 oz. 60
  roasted, chopped or diced, 1 cup 74
slice (Oscar Mayer Jubilee), 1 oz. 14
steak (Oscar Mayer Jubilee), 2 oz. 31

"Ham," vegetarian, frozen:
roll or slices (Worthington Wham) 0

Ham breakfast taco:
(Owens Border Breakfasts), 2.17 oz. 50

Ham dinner, frozen:
(Morton), 10 oz. 45
steak (Armour Classics), 10.75 oz. 50

Ham entrée, frozen:
(Banquet Platters), 10 oz. 50
and asparagus, au gratin (The Budget Gourmet
  Slim Selects), 9 oz. 40

Ham luncheon meat, 1 oz., except as noted:
(Boar's Head Lower Salt) 15
(Healthy Deli Deluxe) 12
(Healthy Deli Lessalt) 13
(Healthy Deli Light AM) 11
(Healthy Deli Taverne) 15
(JM Slice'N Eat 93% Fat Free) 12
(Jones Dairy Farm), 1 slice 21
(Jones Dairy Farm Family Ham) 14
(Oscar Mayer Breakfast Ham), 1.5-oz. slice 21
(Oscar Mayer Jubilee) 15
(Oscar Mayer Lower Salt), .7-oz. slice 10

Ham luncheon meat *(cont.)*
  baked *(Oscar Mayer)*, .7-oz. slice 11
  baked, Virginia *(Healthy Deli)* 12
  Black Forest *(Healthy Deli)* 16
  boiled:
    (Boar's Head Deluxe) 15
    (Oscar Mayer), .7-oz. slice 12
    (Oscar Mayer Thin Sliced), .4-oz. slice 7
  chopped *(Oscar Mayer)* 14
  cooked *(Eckrich Lite)* 15
  cooked, fresh *(Healthy Deli)* 13
  honey:
    (Healthy Deli Honey Valley) 10
    (Oscar Mayer), .7-oz. slice 12
    (Oscar Mayer Thin Sliced), .4-oz. slice 7
  jalapeño *(Healthy Deli)* 11
  minced 20
  pepper, black, cracked *(Oscar Mayer)*, .7-oz. slice 11
  peppered, chopped *(Oscar Mayer)* 16
  smoked, cooked *(Oscar Mayer)*, .7-oz. slice 12
  Virginia *(Healthy Deli* Lessalt) 13

Ham spread, deviled:
  (Underwood), 2 1/8 oz. 50
  (Underwood Light), 2 1/8 oz. 35
  smoked *(Underwood)*, 2 1/8 oz. 65

Ham and cheese loaf:
  (Oscar Mayer), 1 oz. 19

Ham and cheese pocket sandwich, frozen:
  (Hot Pockets), 5 oz. 90

Ham and cheese spread:
  (Oscar Mayer), 1 oz. 15

Hardee's, 1 serving:

Big Country Breakfast:

bacon	305
country ham	345
ham	325
sausage	340
Biscuit 'N' Gravy	15

breakfast biscuit:

bacon	10
bacon and egg	155
bacon, egg, and cheese	165
country ham	25
country ham and egg	175
ham	15
ham and egg	160
ham, egg, and cheese	170
Canadian Rise 'N' Shine	180
chicken	45
Cinnamon 'N' Raisin	0
Rise 'N' Shine	0
sausage	25
sausage and egg	170
steak	30
steak and egg	175
Hash Rounds	0
pancake syrup, 1.5 oz.	0

pancakes, three:

1 serving	15
w/2 bacon strips	25
w/1 sausage patty	40

sandwiches, 1 serving:

Big Deluxe burger	70
Big Roast Beef	45
Big Twin	55
cheeseburger	30
cheeseburger, bacon	80
cheeseburger, 1/4 lb.	70
chicken breast sandwich, grilled	60

Hardee's, sandwiches, 1 serving *(cont.)*

Chicken Fillet	55
Fisherman's Fillet	70
hamburger	20
hot dog, all beef	25
Hot Ham 'N' Cheese	330
Mushroom 'N' Swiss burger	490
roast beef, regular	260
Turkey Club	390

side dishes and special items:

Chicken Stix, 9 piece	55
Chicken Stix, 6 piece	35
Crispy Curls, 3 oz.	0
french fries, large	0
french fries, regular	0

salads:

chef	115
chicken 'N' pasta	55
garden	105
side	0

dressings, 2 oz.:

blue cheese	20
house	25
Thousand Island	35

sauces:

barbecue, 1 pkt.	0
barbecue dipping, 1 oz.	0
Big Twin, .5 oz.	5
honey, .5 oz.	0
sweet mustard dipping, 1 oz.	0
sweet 'n' sour dipping, 1 oz.	0
tartar, .7 oz.	10

desserts and shakes:

apple turnover	0
Big Cookie	5
Cool Twist cone, chocolate, 4.2 oz.	20
Cool Twist cone, vanilla, 4.2 oz.	15
Cool Twist cone, vanilla/chocolate, 4.2 oz.	20

Cool Twist sundae, caramel, 6 oz.	20
Cool Twist sundae, hot fudge, 5.9 oz.	25
Cool Twist sundae, strawberry, 5.9 oz.	15
shake, chocolate, 12 oz.	45
shake, strawberry, 12 oz.	40
shake, vanilla, 12 oz.	50

Hazelnut, see "Filbert"

Head cheese:
(Oscar Mayer), 1 oz.	25

Heart, braised or simmered, 4 oz.:
beef	219
chicken, broiler-fryer	274
lamb	282
pork	251
turkey	256
veal	200

Herb seasoning and coating mix:
Italian *(Shake'n Bake)*	0

Herb side dish mix*:
(Hain)	0

Herbs, see specific listings

Herbs, mixed:
(Lawry's Pinch of Herbs)	0

Herring, fresh, meat only:
Atlantic:
raw, 1 lb.	272
raw, 1 oz.	17
baked, broiled, or microwaved, 4 oz.	87
kippered, 4 oz.	93
pickled, 4 oz.	15

Herring *(cont.)*
   lake, see "Cisco"
   Pacific, raw, 1 lb.   348
   Pacific, raw, 1 oz.   22

Herring, canned, see "Sardine, canned"

Hickory nut:
   dried   0

Hollandaise sauce:
   (Great Impressions), 2 tbsp.   48

Homestyle gravy mix*:
   (French's)   0
   (Pillsbury)   0

Hominy, canned:
   golden or white, plain (all brands)   0

Hominy grits, see "Corn grits"

Honey:
   (all brands)   0

Honey loaf:
   (Oscar Mayer), 1 oz.   16

Honey roll sausage:
   beef, 1 oz.   14

Honeydew:
   fresh   0

Horseradish:
   fresh, leafy tips or pods   0
   prepared, plain or cream style *(Kraft)*   0
   prepared, hot *(Gold's)*   0

The Cholesterol Content of Food

Horseradish sauce:
   (Great Impressions), 1 tbsp.   1
   (Sauceworks), 1 tbsp.   5

Hubbard squash:
   fresh, baked or boiled   0

Hummus:
   dip mix *(Fantastic Foods)*   0
   mix *(Casbah)*   0

Hushpuppy:
   mix, all varieties *(Golden Dipt)*   0

Hyacinth bean:
   fresh or dried   0

I

Food and Measure	Cholesterol (mgs.)
Ice (see also "Sherbet" and "Sorbet"):	
all flavors *(Popsicle/Popsicle* Big Stick)	0
cherry, Italian *(Good Humor)*	0
Ice bar (see also "Fruit bar"), 1 bar:	
all flavors *(Gold Bond* Twin Pop)	0
all flavors *(Good Humor* Ice Stripes)	0
all flavors *(Good Humor Calippo)*	0
all flavors *(Popsicle/Popsicle* Big Stick)	0
Ice cream, 1/2 cup:	
butter almond or butter pecan *(Breyers)*	25
butter crunch *(Sealtest)*	25
butter pecan:	
(Frusen Glädjé)	60

(Häagen-Dazs)	110
(Sealtest)	15
cherry vanilla or chocolate *(Breyers)*	20
chocolate:	
(Frusen Glädjé)	75
(Häagen-Dazs)	120
(Sealtest)	20
mint *(Breyers)*	25
stripes, triple *(Sealtest)*	20
chocolate chip:	
(Dreyer's)	30
(Sealtest)	15
chocolate *(Frusen Glädjé)*	55
chocolate *(Häagen-Dazs)*	105
chocolate, Swiss almond *(Frusen Glädjé)*	55
chocolate marshmallow sundae *(Sealtest)*	20
coffee:	
(Breyers)	30
(Häagen-Dazs)	120
(Sealtest)	15
cookies N' cream *(Breyers)*	20
fudge, marble *(Dreyer's)*	28
fudge royale *(Sealtest)*	15
heavenly hash *(Sealtest)*	15
maple walnut *(Sealtest)*	20
peach *(Breyers)*	15
peanut fudge sundae *(Sealtest)*	20
rocky road *(Dreyer's)*	30
rum raisin *(Häagen-Dazs)*	110
strawberry:	
(Breyers)	20
(Frusen Glädjé)	65
(Häagen-Dazs)	95
(Sealtest)	15
vanilla:	
(Breyers)	25
(Dreyer's)	40
(Frusen Glädjé)	65

Ice cream, vanilla *(cont.)*
  (Häagen-Dazs) 120
  (Sealtest) 20
  French *(Sealtest)* 35
  French, soft-serve 77
  honey *(Häagen-Dazs)* 135
  nuggets, dark chocolate coated *(Carnation Bon
    Bons)*, 5 pieces 14
  nuggets, milk chocolate coated *(Carnation Bon
    Bons)*, 5 pieces 16
  vanilla fudge twirl *(Breyers)* 20
  vanilla peanut butter swirl *(Häagen-Dazs)* 110
  vanilla Swiss almond *(Frusen Glädjé)* 60
  vanilla-chocolate *(Breyers)* 25
  vanilla-chocolate-strawberry:
    (Breyers) 20
    (Sealtest/Sealtest Cubic Scoops) 20
  vanilla-orange *(Sealtest Cubic Scoops)* 15
  vanilla-raspberry *(Sealtest Cubic Scoops)* 15

Ice cream, substitute and imitation, 1/2 cup, except
  as noted:
  all flavors *(Lite-Lite Tofutti/Tofutti)* 0
  all flavors *(Sealtest Free)* 0
  all flavors *(Tofutti Love Drops)* 0
  chocolate *(Simple Pleasures)*, 4 oz. 15
  chocolate chip *(Low, Lite'n Luscious)* 4
  coffee *(Simple Pleasures)*, 4 oz. 15
  Jamoca Swiss almond *(Low, Lite'n Luscious)* 4
  peach *(Simple Pleasures)*, 4 oz. 5
  pineapple coconut *(Low, Lite'n Luscious)* 3
  rum raisin *(Simple Pleasures)*, 4 oz. 10
  strawberry *(Low, Lite'n Luscious)* 3
  strawberry *(Simple Pleasures)*, 4 oz. 11
  vanilla, chocolate dipped *(Tofutti O's)*, 1 piece . . . 0

Ice cream bar, 1 bar:
  (Klondike Lite) 10

caramel almond crunch *(Häagen-Dazs)* 40
chocolate:
   fudge sundae *(Baker's Fudgetastic)* 20
   fudge sundae, crunchy *(Baker's Fudgetastic)* . . . 20
   milk, w/almonds, milk chocolate coated *(Nestlé Premium)* 5
peanut butter crunch *(Häagen-Dazs)* 35
vanilla, white chocolate coated *(Nestlé Alpine)* . . . 5
vanilla crunch *(Häagen-Dazs)* 40

Ice cream bar, substitute and imitation, 1 bar:
all varieties *(Sealtest Free* Dessert Bar) 0
chocolate dip *(Weight Watchers)*, 1.7 oz. 5
chocolate mousse *(Weight Watchers* Sugar Free), 1.75 oz. 5
English toffee crunch *(Weight Watchers)*, 1.7 oz. . . 5
fudge, double *(Weight Watchers)*, 1.75 oz. 5
orange-vanilla treat *(Weight Watchers* Sugar Free), 1.75 oz. 5
vanilla sandwich *(Weight Watchers)*, 2.75 oz. 5

Ice cream cone or cup, plain, 1 piece:
(Little Debbie Ice Cream Cup) . . . . <1

Ice milk, 1/2 cup:
all flavors *(Light n' Lively)* 10
all flavors, except chocolate swirl *(Weight Watchers Grand Collection)* 10
chocolate *(Breyers* Light) 15
chocolate fudge twirl *(Breyers* Light) 10
chocolate swirl *(Weight Watchers Grand Collection)* 5
heavenly hash or praline almond *(Breyers* Light) . . 10
strawberry *(Breyers* Light) 15
toffee fudge parfait or vanilla *(Breyers* Light) 10
vanilla-chocolate-strawberry *(Breyers* Light) 15
vanilla-red raspberry parfait *(Breyers* Light) 15

Icing, cake, see "Frosting"

Italian sausage:
pork, cooked, 1 oz. 22
pork, cooked, 1 link (4 oz. raw) 65

Italian seasoning:
(Tone's) 0

J

Food and Measure	Cholesterol (mgs.)
Jack-in-the-Box, 1 serving:	
breakfast:	
Breakfast Jack	203
crescent, Canadian	226
crescent, sausage	187
crescent, supreme	178
hash browns	3
pancake platter	99
scrambled egg platter	354
sandwiches:	
bacon cheeseburger	85
beef fajita pita	45
cheeseburger	41
cheeseburger, double	72

Jack-in-the-Box, sandwiches *(cont.)*

cheeseburger, ultimate	127
chicken fajita pita	34
chicken fillet, grilled	64
chicken supreme	62
fish supreme	66
hamburger	26
Jumbo Jack	73
Jumbo Jack, w/cheese	102
Swiss and bacon burger	92

Mexican food:

guacamole or salsa	0
taco	21
taco, super	37

salad:

chef	107
Mexican chicken	89
side	<1
taco	92

finger foods:

chicken strips, 4 pieces	68
chicken strips, 6 pieces	103
egg rolls, 3 pieces	30
egg rolls, 5 pieces	50
shrimp, 10 pieces	84
shrimp, 15 pieces	126
taquitos, 5 pieces	37
taquitos, 7 pieces	52

side dishes:

french fries, small	8
french fries, regular	13
onion rings	27

sauces:

BBQ, 1 oz.	0
mayo-mustard, .7 oz.	10
mayo-onion, .7 oz.	20
seafood cocktail, 1 oz.	0
sweet and sour, 1 oz.	<1

dressings, 2.5 oz.:
    bleu cheese 18
    buttermilk 21
    French, reduced calorie 0
    Thousand Island 23
desserts:
    apple turnover 15
    cheesecake 63
shakes, all flavors 25

Jackfruit:
  fresh 0

Jalapeño dip:
  (Kraft), 2 tbsp. 0
  bean *(Wise)*, 2 tbsp. 0
  bean *(Hain)*, 4 tbsp. 5
  cheddar *(Breakstone's* Gourmet), 2 tbsp. 15
  cheese *(Kraft* Premium), 2 tbsp. 15

Jalapeño pepper, see "Pepper, jalapeño"

Jams and jellies:
  all flavors (all brands) 0

Jerusalem artichoke:
  fresh or stored 0

Jicama, see "Yam bean tuber"

Jujube:
  raw or dried 0

Jute, potherb:
  raw or boiled 0

K

Food and Measure	Cholesterol (mgs.)
Kale:	
all varieties, fresh, canned, or frozen	0
Kasha, see "Buckwheat groats"	
Kelp, see "Seaweed"	
Kentucky Fried Chicken:	
chicken, *Original Recipe:*	
breast, center, 4.1 oz.	93
breast, side, 3.2 oz.	77
drumstick, 2 oz.	67
thigh, 3.7 oz.	123
wing, 1.9 oz.	64

The Cholesterol Content of Food

chicken, *Extra Tasty Crispy:*
  breast, center, 4.8 oz. 114
  breast, side, 3.9 oz. 81
  drumstick, 2.4 oz. 71
  thigh, 4.2 oz. 129
  wing, 2.3 oz. 67
chicken, Hot Wings, 6 pieces 148
chicken, *Kentucky Nuggets,* .6 oz. piece 12
chicken, *Lite N' Crispy:*
  breast, center, 3 oz. 57
  breast, side, 2.6 oz. 53
  drumstick, 1.7 oz. 51
  thigh, 2.8 oz. 80
Chicken Littles sandwich, 1.7 oz. 18
Colonel's chicken sandwich, 5.9 oz. 47
Kentucky Nuggets sauces:
  barbecue, mustard, or sweet and sour, 1 oz. . . . <1
  honey, .5 oz. <1
side dishes:
  buttermilk biscuit 1
  coleslaw 5
  corn-on-the-cob . . . . <1
  fries, regular 2
  mashed potatoes, w/gravy, 3.5 oz. . . . . <1

Ketchup, see "Catsup"

Kidney beans, canned:
  red or white, plain (all brands) 0

Kidneys, braised:
  beef, 4 oz. 439
  lamb, 4 oz. 641
  pork, 4 oz. 544
  pork, chopped, 1 cup 673
  veal, 4 oz. 897

Kielbasa (see also "Polish sausage"):
  (Eckrich Lite Polska), 1 oz. 20

Kiwifruit:
  fresh 0

Knockwurst:
  beef *(Hebrew National)*, 1 link 26

Kohlrabi:
  fresh 0

Kumquat:
  fresh 0

L

Food and Measure	Cholesterol (mgs.)
Lamb, choice, meat only, 4 oz., except as noted:	
cubed, leg/shoulder, braised or stewed	122
cubed, leg/shoulder, broiled	102
foreshank, braised:	
lean w/fat	120
lean w/fat, diced, 1 cup, 4.9 oz.	148
lean only	118
lean only, diced, 1 cup, 4.9 oz.	146
ground:	
raw, 1 oz.	21
broiled	110
broiled, 1 cup	113
leg, whole, roasted:	
lean w/fat	105

Lamb, leg, whole, roasted *(cont.)*
    lean w/fat, 1 slice, 3″ diam. × 1/4″ 26
    lean only 101
    lean only, 3″-diam. slice 25
  leg, shank, roasted:
    lean w/fat 102
    lean w/fat, 1 slice, 3″ diam. × 1/4″ 26
    lean only 99
    lean only, 3″-diam. slice 25
  leg, sirloin, roasted:
    lean w/fat 110
    lean w/fat, 1 slice, 3″ diam. × 1/4″ 27
    lean only 104
    lean only, 3″-diam. slice 26
  loin chop, broiled:
    lean w/fat, 2.25 oz. (4.2 oz. raw w/bone) 64
    lean w/fat 113
    lean only, 1.6 oz. (4.2 oz. raw w/bone and fat) . . 44
    lean only 108
  loin, roasted, lean w/fat 108
  loin, roasted, lean only 99
  rib:
    broiled, lean w/fat 112
    broiled, lean only 103
    roasted, lean w/fat 110
    roasted, lean only 100
  shoulder, whole:
    braised, lean w/fat 132
    braised, lean only 133
    roasted, lean w/fat 104
    roasted, lean only 99

Lamb, New Zealand, frozen, meat only, 4 oz.,
  except as noted:
  foreshank, braised, lean w/fat 116
  foreshank, braised, lean only 115
  leg, whole, roasted, lean w/fat 115
  leg, whole, roasted, lean only 113

The Cholesterol Content of Food

loin chop, broiled:
lean w/fat, 1.5 oz. (3 oz. raw w/bone)   48
lean w/fat. 127
lean only, 1.1 oz. (3 oz. raw w/bone and fat) . . .   34
lean only 129
rib, roasted, lean w/fat 113
rib, roasted, lean only 107
shoulder, braised, lean w/fat 139
shoulder, braised, lean only 144

Lamb's-quarters:
raw or cooked   0

Lard, pork:
1 tbsp.   12

Lasagna dinner, frozen:
(Banquet Extra Helping), 16.5 oz.   38

Lasagna entrée, canned or packaged:
(Chef Boyardee Microwave), 7.5 oz.   18
in garden vegetable sauce *(Chef Boyardee*
Microwave), 7.5 oz.   3
Italian *(Hormel Top Shelf),* 1 serving   40
vegetable *(Hormel Top Shelf),* 10.6 oz.   35

Lasagna entrée, frozen:
cheese *(Dining Lite),* 9 oz.   30
cheese, Italian *(Weight Watchers),* 11 oz.   30
cheese, three *(The Budget Gourmet),* 10 oz.   65
garden *(Weight Watchers),* 11 oz.   20
meat *(Buitoni* Single Serving), 9 oz. 110
w/meat sauce:
(The Budget Gourmet Slim Selects), 10 oz.   25
(Dining Lite), 9 oz.   25
(Healthy Choice), 9 oz.   20
(Le Menu LightStyle), 10 oz.   30
(Weight Watchers), 11 oz.   45

Lasagna entrée, frozen *(cont.)*
in sauce *(Buitoni* Family Style), 7.3 oz. 55
sausage, Italian *(The Budget Gourmet)*, 10 oz. . . . 80
seafood *(Mrs. Paul's* Light), 9.5 oz. 57
w/tofu *(Legume* Classic), 8 oz. 0
tuna, w/spinach noodles and vegetables *(Lean
Cuisine)*, 9.75 oz. 35
vegetable, garden *(Le Menu* LightStyle), 10.5 oz. . . 25
vegetable, w/tofu *(Legume)*, 12 oz. 0
zucchini *(Lean Cuisine)*, 11 oz. 25

Leek:
fresh or freeze-dried 0

Lemon:
fresh 0

Lemon butter dill cooking sauce:
(Golden Dipt) 0

Lemon dill seasoning:
(McCormick/Schilling Bag'n Season) 0

Lemon drink:
(all brands) 0

Lemon extract:
(Virginia Dare) 0

Lemon-herb marinade:
(Golden Dipt) 0

Lemon juice:
fresh, canned, or frozen 0

Lemon peel:
fresh or dried 0

Lemon pepper seasoning:
(Lawry's) 0
(McCormick/Schilling Parsley Patch) 0
(McCormick/Schilling Spice Blends) 0

Lemon-lime drink:
(all brands) 0

Lemonade:
canned, chilled, frozen, or mix (all brands) 0

Lentil:
all varieties 0

Lentil pilaf mix:
(Casbah) 0

Lentil rice loaf, frozen:
(Harvest Bake) 0

Lentil sprouts:
fresh 0

Lettuce:
all varieties 0

Lima beans:
fresh, canned, or frozen, w/out sauce 0
frozen, in butter sauce *(Green Giant),* 1/2 cup 5
frozen, in butter sauce *(Stokely Singles),* 4 oz. . . . 5

Lima beans, mature:
baby or large, dry or canned 0

Lime:
fresh 0

Lime juice:
fresh, reconstituted, or sweetened 0

Limeade, frozen:
  (all brands)   0

Ling cod, meat only:
  raw, 1 lb.   236
  raw, 1 oz.   15

Linguine, see "Pasta"

Linguine entrée, frozen:
  w/scallops and clams *(The Budget Gourmet),*
    9.5 oz.   60
  w/shrimp *(The Budget Gourmet),* 10 oz.   75
  w/shrimp *(Healthy Choice),* 9.5 oz.   55

Linguine entrée, packaged:
  w/clam sauce *(Hormel Top Shelf),* 1 serving   85

Liquor, pure distilled:
  all varieties, all proofs   0

Little Caesars, 1 serving:
  Caesars Sandwich:
    ham and cheese   45
    Italian sub   60
    tuna melt   65
    vegetarian   55
  pizza:
    cheese, single slice   10
    cheese, w/salad   35
    combination, single slice   15
    combination, w/salad   40
  salad, w/low-calorie dressing:
    antipasto, 12 oz.   40
    Greek, 11 oz.   25
    tossed, 11 oz.   0

Liver:
  beef, pan-fried, 4 oz.   547

chicken, simmered, 4 oz. 716
chicken, simmered, chopped, 1 cup 883
duck, raw, 1 oz. 146
lamb, pan-fried, 4 oz. 559
pork, braised, 4 oz. 403
turkey, simmered, 4 oz. 710
turkey, simmered, chopped, 1 cup 876
veal (calves'), braised, 4 oz. 636
veal (calves'), pan-fried, 4 oz. 374

Liver cheese:
(Oscar Mayer), 1.34-oz. slice 80

Liver pâté, see "Pâté"

Liverwurst (see also "Braunschweiger"):
(Jones Dairy Farm), 1 slice 43
(Jones Dairy Farm Chub), 1 oz. 43

Liverwurst spread:
(Underwood), 2 1/8 oz. 90

Lobster, northern, meat only:
raw, 1 oz. 27
boiled or steamed, 4 oz. 82
boiled or steamed, 1 cup 104

Lobster, spiny, see "Spiny lobster"

Lobster sauce, canned:
rock *(Progresso)*, 1/2 cup 10

Loganberry:
fresh or frozen 0

Longan, shelled:
fresh or dried 0

Loquat:
   fresh 0

Lotte, see "Monkfish"

Lotus root or seed:
   raw, dried, or cooked 0

Lox, see "Salmon, Chinook"

Luncheon meat (see also specific listings):
   (Oscar Mayer), 1-oz. slice 21

Luncheon "meat," vegetarian, canned:
   (Worthington Numete/Protose) 0

Lupin:
   boiled 0

Lychee:
   raw or dried 0

M

Food and Measure	Cholesterol (mgs.)
Macadamia nut:	
dried or oil-roasted	0
Macaroni (see also "Noodle" listings and "Pasta"):	
all types, except egg, dry or cooked, plain	0
Macaroni dishes, canned or packaged:	
and beef *(Chef Boyardee Beefaroni Microwave),*	
7.5 oz.	18
and cheese *(Hormel Micro-Cup),* 7.5 oz.	17
elbows, w/beef sauce *(Chef Boyardee Microwave),*	
7.5 oz.	15
shells and cheddar *(Lipton Hearty Ones),* 11 oz. . .	14

Macaroni and cheese dinner, frozen:
(Banquet), 10 oz.	30
w/mini franks *(Kid Cuisine)*, 9 oz.	40

Macaroni and cheese dishes, frozen:
(The Budget Gourmet Side Dish), 5.3 oz.	25
(Green Giant One Serving), 5.7 oz.	25

Macaroni and cheese dishes, mix:
(Golden Grain Macaroni & Cheddar), 1.81 oz.	4
(Kraft/Kraft Family Size Dinner), 3/4 cup*	5
(Kraft Deluxe Dinner), 3/4 cup*	20
shells *(Velveeta* Dinner), 1/2 cup*	20
shells *(Velveeta* Touch of Mexico), 1/2 cup*	20
spirals *(Kraft* Dinner), 3/4 cup*	10
w/bacon, shells *(Velveeta* Bits Of Bacon), 1/2 cup*	25

Mace, ground:
(all brands)	0

Mackerel, fresh, meat only:
Atlantic:
raw, 1 lb.	318
raw, 1 oz.	20
baked, broiled, or microwaved, 4 oz.	85
king, raw, 1 lb.	242
king, raw, 1 oz.	15
Pacific and jack, raw, 1 lb.	213
Pacific and jack, raw, 1 oz.	13

Spanish:
raw, 1 lb.	345
raw, 1 oz.	22
baked, broiled, or microwaved, 4 oz.	83

Mackerel, canned:
jack, drained, 4 oz.	90

Mahi mahi, see "Dolphin fish"

Mai tai mix:
bottled or instant *(Holland House)* 0

Mammy apple:
fresh 0

Mango:
fresh 0

Mango nectar:
(Libby's) 0

Manhattan cocktail mix:
bottled *(Holland House)* 0

Manicotti entrée, frozen:
(Buitoni Single Serving), 9 oz. 130
cheese *(Weight Watchers)*, 9.25 oz. 75
cheese, w/meat sauce *(The Budget Gourmet)*,
10 oz. 50
w/spinach and tofu *(Legume* Florentine), 11 oz. . . . 0
w/tofu *(Legume* Classic), 8 oz. 0

Maple sugar, see "Sugar, maple"

Maple syrup:
(all brands) 0

Margarine:
plain, stick, soft, spread, squeeze, or whipped (all
brands) 0
spread *(Kraft "Touch of Butter")*, 1 tbsp. 0

Margarita cocktail mix:
bottled, all flavors *(Holland House)* 0

Marinade, see specific listings

Marjoram, dried:
(all brands) 0

Marmalade:
all flavors (all brands) 0

Marrow squash:
fresh 0

Marshmallow topping:
(Marshmallow Fluff) 0
creme *(Kraft)* 0

Matzo crumbs and meal:
all varieties *(Manischewitz)* 0

Mayonnaise (see also "Salad dressing"), 1 tbsp.:
(Cains) 10
(Hain Light Low Sodium) 10
(Hellmann's/Best Foods) 5
(Hellmann's/Best Foods Light) 5
(Kraft Real) 5
(Kraft Light) 0
(Rokeach) 10
(Weight Watchers Reduced Calorie) 5
canola, reduced calorie *(Hain)* 5
cholesterol free *(Hellmann's)* 0
cold processed, canola, eggless, real, or safflower
(Hain) 5
regular, canola, or safflower *(Hollywood)* 5
soy *(Featherweight Soyamaise)* 5
tofu *(Nasoya Nayonaise)* 0

McDonald's, 1 serving:
breakfast dishes:
eggs, scrambled 399
hashbrown potatoes 9
hotcakes, w/butter and syrup 21

sausage, pork 48
breakfast biscuit or sandwich:
  w/bacon, egg, and cheese 253
  w/biscuit spread 1
  Egg McMuffin 226
  w/sausage 49
  w/sausage and egg 275
  Sausage McMuffin 64
  Sausage McMuffin, w/egg 263
danish:
  apple 25
  cinnamon raisin 34
  iced cheese 47
  raspberry 26

muffin:
  apple bran 0
  English, w/butter 9

sandwiches and chicken:
  Big Mac 103
  cheeseburger 53
  Chicken McNuggets 65
  Filet-O-Fish 50
  hamburger 37
  McChicken 43
  McD.L.T. 109
  McLean Deluxe, 7.3 oz. 60
  McLean Deluxe (patty only), 3 oz. 60
  McLean Deluxe, w/cheese, 7.7 oz. 75
  Quarter Pounder 86
  Quarter Pounder, w/cheese 118
french fries, medium 12
salads:
  chef 128
  chunky chicken 78
  garden 83
  side 41

McDonald's *(cont.)*
  salad dressing, 1/5 pkg.:
    blue cheese 6
    peppercorn 7
    Thousand Island 8
  sauces, 1 serving:
    barbecue, honey, or sweet and sour 0
    hot mustard 5
  pies and cookies:
    apple pie 6
    cookies, chocolaty chip 4
    cookies, *McDonaldland* 0
  shakes, lowfat, all flavors 10
  yogurt, frozen, lowfat:
    cone, vanilla 3
    sundae, hot caramel 13
    sundae, hot fudge 6
    sundae, strawberry 5

Meat, see specific listings

"Meat" loaf, vegetarian, mix*:
  (Natural Touch) 0

Meat loaf dinner, frozen:
  (Armour Classics), 11.25 oz. 65
  (Banquet), 11 oz. 85
  (Morton), 10 oz. 50

Meat marinade mix:
  (French's) 0

"Meatball," vegetarian, canned:
  (Worthington Non-Meat Balls) 0

Meatball dinner, frozen:
  Swedish *(Armour Classics)*, 11.25 oz. 80

The Cholesterol Content of Food

Meatball entrée, frozen:

Italian style *(The Budget Gourmet)*, 10 oz.	55
stew *(Lean Cuisine)*, 10 oz.	85
Swedish, w/noodles *(The Budget Gourmet)*, 10 oz.	140
Swedish, w/pasta and vegetables *(Le Menu LightStyle)*, 8 oz.	40
Swedish, sauce and *(Dining Lite)*, 9 oz.	55

Melon balls, frozen:

cantaloupe and honeydew	0

Menudo, canned:

(Old El Paso), 1/2 can	176

Mesquite sauce:

w/lime juice *(Lawry's)*	0

Mesquite seasoning:

(Tone's)	0

Mexican beans, canned:

(Old El Paso Mexe-Beans)	0

Mexican dinner, frozen (see also specific listings):

(Patio Fiesta), 12.25 oz.	30
style *(Morton)*, 10 oz.	20
style *(Patio)*, 13.25 oz.	45

Mexican seasoning:

(Tone's), 1 tsp.	tr.

Milk, cow, fluid, 1 cup:

buttermilk, cultured	9
buttermilk, lowfat 1.5%, unsalted *(Friendship)*	14
whole, 3.7% fat, producer	35
whole, 3.3% fat	33
lowfat:	
2% fat, plain or nonfat milk solids added	18

Milk, lowfat *(cont.)*

    2% fat, protein fortified 19

    1% fat, plain, nonfat milk solids added, or

       protein fortified 10

  skim 4

  skim, nonfat milk solids added or protein fortified   5

Milk, canned:

  condensed, sweetened, 1 cup 104

  condensed, sweetened, 1 tbsp. 6

  evaporated:

    whole, 1 cup 73

    whole, 1 tbsp. 5

    skim, 1 cup 10

    skim, 1 tbsp. . . . . <1

    skim *(Pet Light)*, 1/2 cup 5

    filled *(Pet/Dairymate)*, 1/2 cup 5

    imitation, filled *(Diehl)*, 1/2 cup 5

Milk, chocolate, see "Chocolate milk"

Milk, dry:

  buttermilk, sweet cream, 1 cup 83

  buttermilk, sweet cream, 1 tbsp. 5

  whole, 1 cup 124

  nonfat:

    regular, 1 cup 24

    instant, 1 cup 17

    instant, 3.2-oz. envelope or 1 1/3 cup 12

    instant *(Carnation)*, 5 level tbsp. 5

    instant *(Sanalac* Dairy Fresh), .8 oz. 5

Milk, goats:

  whole, 1 cup 28

Milk, imitation:

  fluid, 1 cup . . . . tr.

  soy, see "Soy milk"

The Cholesterol Content of Food

Milk beverages, see specific flavors

Milkfish, meat only:
raw, 1 lb.	235
raw, 1 oz.	15

Milkshake, frozen:
chocolate or strawberry *(MicroMagic)*, 11.5 oz.	40
vanilla *(MicroMagic)*, 11.5 oz.	45

Millet:
raw or cooked	0

Mincemeat, see "Pie filling, canned"

Miso:
all varieties	0

Molasses:
all varieties (all brands)	0

Monkfish, meat only:
raw, 1 lb.	115
raw, 1 oz.	7

Monosodium glutamate:
(Tone's)	0

Mortadella:
beef and pork, 1 oz.	16

Mothbean:
boiled	0

Mother's loaf:
pork, 1 oz.	13

Mousse, see specific listings

Muffin, 1 piece, except as noted:

all varieties *(Wonder)*	0
apple or apple streusel *(Awrey's)*	35
banana nut *(Awrey's)*	30
banana-walnut or blueberry, mini *(Hostess Breakfast Bake Shop)*, 5 pieces	40
blueberry *(Awrey's)*	20
cinnamon apple, mini *(Hostess Breakfast Bake Shop)*, 5 pieces	45
corn *(Awrey's)*	25
cranberry *(Awrey's)*	10
English:	
(Roman Meal Original)	0
all varieties *(Hi Fiber)*	0
all varieties *(Oatmeal Goodness)*	0
all varieties *(Pepperidge Farm)*	0
all varieties *(Thomas')*	0
oat bran, all varieties *(Awrey's)*	0
oat bran, all varieties *(Hostess Breakfast Bake Shop)*	0
raisin-bran *(Awrey's)*	20

Muffin, frozen, 1 piece:

all varieties *(Sara Lee)*	0
banana nut *(Weight Watchers)*, 2.5 oz.	10
blueberry:	
(Pepperidge Farm Old Fashioned)	25
(Sara Lee Free & Light)	0
(Weight Watchers), 2.5 oz.	10
corn *(Pepperidge Farm* Old Fashioned)	30
oat bran w/apple or raisin bran *(Pepperidge Farm* Old Fashioned)	0

Muffin, mix*, 1 piece:

apple cinnamon, blackberry, or blueberry *(Martha White)*	3
bran *(Martha White)*	14
oat bran, all varieties *(Hain)*	0

orangeberry *(Martha White)* 2
raspberry or strawberry *(Martha White)* 3

Mulberry:
fresh 0

Mullet, striped, meat only:
raw, 1 lb. 224
raw, 1 oz. 14
baked, broiled, or microwaved, 4 oz. 71

Mung beans:
boiled 0

Mungo beans:
boiled 0

Mushroom:
all varieties, fresh, canned, dried, or frozen, plain . . 0
frozen, battered *(Stilwell Quickkrisp)*, 2 oz. 5

Mushroom and herb dip:
(Breakstone's Gourmet), 2 tbsp. 10

Mussel, blue, meat only:
raw, 1 oz. 8
raw, 1 cup 42
boiled or steamed, 4 oz. 64

Mustard, prepared:
all varieties (all brands) 0

Mustard greens:
fresh, canned, or frozen 0

Mustard powder:
(all brands) 0

Mustard seed:
  yellow 0

Mustard spinach:
  fresh 0

Mustard tallow:
  1 tbsp. 13

N

Food and Measure	Cholesterol (mgs.)
Natto:	
all varieties	0
Navy beans:	
raw or canned	0
Nectarine:	
fresh	0
New England Brand Sausage:	
(Oscar Mayer), .8-oz. slice	14
New Zealand spinach:	
fresh	0

Noodle, Chinese:
cellophane, long rice, or chow mein 0

Noodle, egg:
uncooked, 2 oz.:
  (Creamette) 70
  (Golden Grain) 65
  (Mueller's) 55
  (Prince) 65
cooked, 1 cup 53
cooked, spinach, 1 cup 52

Noodle, Japanese:
soba, somen, or udon 0

Noodle and chicken dinner, frozen:
(Banquet), 10 oz. 45
(Banquet Family Favorites), 10 oz. 45

Noodle and chicken entrée, packaged:
(Hormel/Dinty Moore Micro-Cup), 7.5 oz. 20

Noodle dishes, mix*, 1/2 cup, except as noted:
Alfredo *(Minute* Microwave Family Size) 45
Alfredo *(Minute* Microwave Single Size) 40
cheese *(Kraft* Dinner), 3/4 cup 50
chicken or chicken flavor:
  (Kraft Dinner), 3/4 cup 45
  (Minute Microwave Family/Single Size) 35
  and mushroom *(Golden Grain/Noodle Roni),*
    1.2 oz. dry 19
fettuccine *(Golden Grain/Noodle Roni),* 1.5 oz. dry 27
garlic, creamy *(Golden Grain/Noodle Roni),* 1.5 oz.
  dry 29
herb and butter or Parmesano *(Golden Grain/
  Noodle Roni),* 1 oz. dry 19
Parmesan *(Minute* Microwave Family Size) 45
Parmesan *(Minute* Microwave Single Size) 40

Romanoff *(Golden Grain/Noodle Roni)*, 1.5 oz. dry   23
Stroganoff *(Golden Grain/Noodle Roni)*, 2 oz. dry . .   42

Nut topping:
(Planters)   0

Nutmeg:
ground (all brands)   0

Nuts, see specific listings

Nuts, mixed:
all varieties (all brands)   0

O

Food and Measure	Cholesterol (mgs.)
Oat (see also ''Cereal''):	
whole-grain, flakes, rolled, or oatmeal	0
Oat bran:	
raw or cooked	0
Oat flour:	
whole-grain or blend	0
Ocean perch:	
fresh, Atlantic, meat only:	
raw, 1 lb.	191
raw, 1 oz.	12
baked, broiled, or microwaved, 4 oz.	61
frozen *(Van de Kamp's* Natural), 4 oz.	40

The Cholesterol Content of Food

Ocean perch entrée, frozen:
(Van de Kamp's Light), 1 piece   35

Octopus, meat only:
raw, 1 lb.   219
raw, 1 oz.   14

Oheloberry:
fresh   0

Oil:
almond, avocado, cocoa butter, coconut, corn,
     cottonseed, hazelnut, mustard, nutmeg butter,
     olive, palm, palm kernel, peanut, poppyseed,
     safflower, sesame, soybean, sunflower,
     vegetable, or walnut   0
cod liver, regular or mint flavor (Hain), 1 tbsp.   85
cod liver, cherry flavor (Hain), 1 tbsp.   75

Okra:
fresh or frozen, w/out sauce   0

Old-fashioned cocktail mix:
bottled (Holland House)   0

Old-fashioned loaf:
(Oscar Mayer), 1 oz.   16

Olive, pickled:
green or ripe, all varieties, all sizes   0

Olive appetizer:
(Progresso/Progresso Condite)   0

Olive loaf:
(Boar's Head), 1 oz.   10
(Oscar Mayer), 1 oz.   8

Onion, mature:
  fresh, canned, dried, or frozen, w/out sauce   0
  frozen, w/cream sauce, small *(Birds Eye*
     Combinations), 5 oz.   0

Onion, green (scallion):
  fresh   0

Onion, Welsh:
  fresh   0

Onion dip:
  bean *(Hain)*, 4 tbsp.   5
  creamy, plain or French *(Kraft Premium)*, 2 tbsp. . . .   10
  French:
    (Bison), 1 oz.   20
    (Breakstone's/Sealtest), 2 tbsp.   15
    (Nasoya Vegi-Dip), 1 oz.   0
  French or green *(Kraft)*, 2 tbsp.   0
  toasted *(Breakstone's* Gourmet), 2 tbsp.   10

Onion-flavor snack:
  (Funyuns)   0
  rings *(Wise)*   0

Onion powder:
  (all brands)   0

Onion rings, frozen:
  (Ore-Ida Onion Ringers), 2 oz.   0
  battered *(Stilwell)*, 3 oz. . . . .   <1
  crispy *(Farm Rich Onion O's)*, 5 rings   0

Onion salt:
  (all brands)   0

Orange:
  all varieties, fresh or canned   0

The Cholesterol Content of Food

Orange drink:
   (all brands)   0

Orange extract:
   (Virginia Dare)   0

Orange juice or juice drink:
   fresh, canned, or frozen   0
   blends (all brands)   0

Orange sauce:
   mandarin *(La Choy)*   0

Oregano:
   fresh or dried (all brands)   0

Oriental 5-spice:
   (Tone's)   0

Oyster, meat only:
   fresh, Eastern:
      raw, 1 lb.   248
      raw, 6 medium, 3 oz.   46
      steamed or poached, 4 oz.   124
   canned, Eastern, w/liquid, 4 oz.   62

Oyster stew, see "Soup, canned, condensed"

P

Food and Measure	Cholesterol (mgs.)
Pancake, frozen:	
blueberry *(Aunt Jemima* Microwave), 3.5 oz.	21
buttermilk *(Aunt Jemima* Microwave), 3.5 oz.	20
buttermilk *(Weight Watchers),* 2.5 oz.	10
Pancake batter, frozen:	
(Aunt Jemima Original), 3.6 oz.	19
blueberry or buttermilk *(Aunt Jemima),* 3.6 oz.	27
Pancake breakfast, frozen:	
w/blueberry topping *(Weight Watchers),* 4.75 oz.	10
w/links *(Weight Watchers),* 4 oz.	15
w/strawberry topping *(Weight Watchers),* 4.75 oz.	10

Pancake and waffle mix*, 3 pieces, 4″ each:
(Aunt Jemima Original) 0
(Aunt Jemima Original Complete) 16
all varieties *(Bisquick Shake'N Pour)* 0
buttermilk *(Aunt Jemima)* 1
buttermilk *(Aunt Jemima* Complete) 9
whole wheat *(Aunt Jemima)* 0

Pancake syrup:
(Vermont Maid) 0
all varieties *(Aunt Jemima)* 0
all varieties *(Log Cabin)* 0

Pancreas, braised:
lamb, 4 oz. 454
pork, 4 oz. 357

Papaya:
fresh 0

Papaya nectar:
(Libby's) 0

Papaya punch:
(Veryfine) 0

Paprika:
all varieties (all brands) 0

Parsley:
fresh or dried 0

Parsley root:
1 oz. 0

Parsley seasoning:
all purpose *(McCormick/Schilling Parsley Patch)* . . 0

Parsnip:
   raw or cooked   0

Passion fruit:
   all varieties, fresh   0

Passion fruit juice:
   all varieties and blends (all brands)   0

Pasta, dry (see also "Macaroni" and "Noodle"
listings):
   dry:
      all varieties, except w/egg (all brands)   0
      corn, wheat-free *(De Boles)*   0
      w/egg *(Creamette)*, 2 oz. 70
      spinach, w/egg *(Creamette)*, 2 oz. 70
   cooked, all varieties, except w/egg   0

Pasta, fresh-refrigerated:
   w/egg, uncooked, regular or spinach, 2 oz. 41
   w/egg, cooked, regular or spinach, 4 oz. 37

Pasta dinner, frozen, see specific listings

Pasta dishes, canned (see also specific listings):
   in cheese-flavored sauce *(Chef Boyardee* ABC's/
      123's/Dinosaurs Microwave), 7.5 oz.   3
   in cheese-flavored sauce *(Chef Boyardee* Tic Tac
      Toes Microwave), 7.5 oz.   2
   garden medley *(Lipton Hearty Ones)*, 11 oz.   6
   w/meatballs *(Chef Boyardee* ABC's/123's/
      Dinosaurs Microwave), 7.5 oz. 17
   w/meatballs *(Chef Boyardee* Tic Tac Toes
      Microwave), 7.5 oz. 16
   w/meatballs, in sauce, rings or twists *(Buitoni)*,
      7.5 oz. 20
   rings, in sauce *(Buitoni)*, 7.5 oz.   5
   shells, in meat sauce *(Chef Boyardee* Microwave),
      7.5 oz. 15

shells, in mushroom sauce *(Chef Boyardee
Microwave)*, 7.5 oz.   2
twists, in sauce *(Buitoni)*, 7.5 oz.   0

Pasta dishes, frozen (see also "Pasta entree" and
specific listings):
all varieties *(Green Giant Pasta Accents)*, 1/2 cup . .   5
Alfredo, w/broccoli *(The Budget Gourmet Side
Dish)*, 5.5 oz.   25
Dijon *(Green Giant Garden Gourmet)*, 1 pkg.   55
Florentine *(Green Giant Garden Gourmet)*, 1 pkg.   25
marinara *(Green Giant One Serving)*, 5.5 oz.   0
Parmesan, w/sweet peas *(Green Giant One
Serving)*, 5.5 oz.   10
shells and beef *(The Budget Gourmet)*, 10 oz. . . .   35
and vegetables, w/out added ingredients:
in Stroganoff sauce *(Birds Eye Custom Cuisine)*,
4.6 oz.   30
in white cheese sauce *(Birds Eye Custom
Cuisine)*, 4.6 oz.   15

Pasta dishes, mix* (see also specific listings),
1/2 cup, except as noted:
(Kraft Light Rancher's Choice Pasta Salad)   0
(McCormick/Schilling Pasta Prima), 1 pkg. dry . . .   0
w/bacon *(Kraft Light Rancher's Choice Pasta
Salad)*   10
broccoli and vegetables *(Kraft Pasta Salad)*   10
cheddar:
(Minute Microwave Family/Single Size)   15
broccoli *(Kraft Pasta & Cheese)*   30
tangy *(Hain Pasta & Sauce)*, 1/4 pkg.   3
chicken w/herbs *(Kraft Pasta & Cheese)*   25
fettuccine Alfredo *(Kraft Pasta & Cheese)*   30
homestyle *(Kraft Pasta Salad)*   10
Italian *(Kraft Light Pasta Salad)*   0
Parmesan *(Kraft Pasta & Cheese)*   30
Parmesan, creamy *(Hain Pasta & Sauce)*, 1/4 pkg.   10

Pasta dishes, mix* *(cont.)*
  primavera *(Hain* Pasta & Sauce), 1/4 pkg. 10
  primavera, garden *(Kraft* Pasta Salad) 0
  sour cream and chives *(Kraft* Pasta & Cheese) . . . 25
  three cheese w/vegetables *(Kraft* Pasta & Cheese) 25

Pasta entrée, frozen (see also specific listings):
  angel hair *(Weight Watchers),* 10 oz. 20
  primavera *(Weight Watchers),* 8.5 oz. 5
  rigati *(Weight Watchers),* 10.63 oz. 25

Pasta sauce, canned (see also specific listings):
  (Progresso Spaghetti Sauce), 1/2 cup 2
  all varieties *(Enrico's* All Natural), 4 oz. 0
  all varieties *(Ragu),* 4 oz. 0
  marinara *(Buitoni)* 0
  marinara *(Prego),* 4 oz. 0
  marinara *(Progresso),* 1/2 cup 1
  marinara *(Progresso* Authentic Pasta Sauces),
    1/2 cup 4
  meat flavor *(Progresso* Spaghetti Sauce), 1/2 cup . . 5
  mushroom *(Progresso* Spaghetti Sauce), 1/2 cup . . 5
  primavera, creamy *(Progresso* Authentic Pasta
    Sauces), 1/2 cup 54
  Sicilian *(Progresso* Authentic Pasta Sauces),
    1/2 cup 0
  traditional or mushroom flavor *(Hunt's),* 4 oz. 0

Pasta sauce, refrigerated (see also specific listings):
  marinara *(Contadina Fresh),* 7.5 oz. 0
  plum, w/basil *(Contadina Fresh),* 7.5 oz. 5

Pastrami:
  (Boar's Head), 1 oz. 16
  (Healthy Deli), 1 oz. 14
  (Oscar Mayer), .6-oz. slice 7
  turkey, see "Turkey pastrami"

Pastry shell (see also "Pie crust shell"):
  pocket *(Pillsbury),* 1 piece 0
  tart shell *(Pet-Ritz),* 1 piece 7

Pâté, canned:
   (Sells Liver Pâté), 2 1/8 oz. 90
   goose liver, smoked, 1 oz. 43
   goose liver, smoked, 1 tbsp. 20

Pea pods, Chinese, see "Peas, edible-podded"

Peach:
   fresh, canned, dried, or frozen 0

Peach butter:
   (Smuckers) 0

Peach drink or juice:
   (all brands) 0

Peach nectar:
   (Libby's) 0

Peanut:
   all varieties (all brands) 0

Peanut butter:
   all varieties (all brands) 0

Peanut butter flavor baking chips:
   (Reese's), 1/4 cup 5

Peanut butter-caramel topping:
   (Smucker's) 0

Peanut flour:
   defatted or lowfat 0

Peanut oil, see "Oil"

Pear:
   fresh, canned, or dried 0

Pear nectar:
canned   0

Peas, see specific listings

Peas, cream, canned:
(Allens)   0

Peas, crowder:
canned or frozen, plain (all brands)   0

Peas, edible-podded:
fresh or frozen, all varieties   0

Peas, field:
canned, all varieties   0

Peas, green or sweet:
fresh, canned, or frozen, w/out sauce   0
frozen in butter sauce:
   early *(Green Giant* One Serving), 4.5 oz.   5
   early *(LeSueur),* 1/2 cup   5
   sweet *(Green Giant),* 1/2 cup   5
   sweet *(Stokely Singles),* 4 oz.   5
frozen, w/cream sauce *(Birds Eye* Combinations),
  5 oz.   0

Peas, green, combinations, frozen:
and carrots, w/out sauce (all brands)   0
and cauliflower, in cream sauce *(The Budget
Gourmet* Side Dish), 5.75 oz.   20
w/pearl onions, in cheese sauce *(Birds Eye* Cheese
Sauce Combinations), 5 oz.   5
and potatoes, w/cream sauce *(Birds Eye*
Combinations), 5 oz.   0
and water chestnuts Oriental *(The Budget
Gourmet),* 5 oz.   5

The Cholesterol Content of Food

Peas, purple hull:
canned or frozen   0

Peas, sprouted, mature seeds:
raw or boiled   0

Peas, white acre:
canned, fresh *(Allens)*   0

Pecan:
dried, dry-roasted, or oil-roasted   0

Pecan flour:
1 cup   0

Pecan topping:
in syrup *(Smucker's)*   0

Pepper, ground:
all varieties and blends (all brands)   0

Pepper, bell, see "Pepper, sweet"

Pepper, cherry:
mild *(Vlasic)*   0

Pepper, chili:
green or red, fresh or canned   0

Pepper, jalapeño:
all styles (all brands)   0

Pepper, pepperoncini:
salad *(Vlasic)*   0

Pepper, sweet:
fresh, freeze-dried, or frozen, green and red   0
in jars, roasted or fried *(Progresso)*   0

Pepper rings:
hot *(Vlasic)* 0

Pepper sauce, hot:
(Gebhardt Louisiana Style) 0
(Tabasco) 0

Peppered loaf:
(Oscar Mayer), 1 oz. 14

Pepperoni:
(Hickory Farms) 23

Perch, meat only (see also "Ocean perch"):
raw, 1 lb. 407
raw, 1 oz. 26
baked, broiled, or microwaved, 4 oz. 130

Perch entrée, frozen:
battered *(Van de Kamp's)*, 2 pieces 30

Persimmon:
Japanese or native, fresh 0

Pesto sauce:
refrigerated *(Contadina Fresh)*, 2 1/3 oz. 10

Picante sauce (see also "Salsa"):
(Gebhardt), 1 tbsp. 0
(Old El Paso), 2 tbsp. 0
(Pace), 2 tsp. 0
(Wise), 2 tbsp. 0
mild *(Azteca)*, 1 tbsp. 0

Pickle:
all varieties (all brands) 0

Pickle and pimiento loaf:
(Oscar Mayer), 1 oz. 13

Picnic loaf:
  (Oscar Mayer), 1 oz.   16

Pie, frozen:
  all varieties *(Sara Lee Free & Light)*, 1/8 pie   0
  all varieties, except pecan and pumpkin *(Mrs. Smith's "Pie In Minutes")*, 1/8 pie   0
  all varieties, except pecan and pumpkin *(Sara Lee Homestyle)*, 1/10 of 9″ pie   0
  apple *(Weight Watchers)*, 3.5 oz.   5
  Boston cream, see "Cake, frozen"
  chocolate mocha *(Weight Watchers)*, 2.75 oz.   5
  pecan or pumpkin *(Mrs. Smith's "Pie In Minutes")*, 1/8 pie   35
  pecan *(Sara Lee Homestyle)*, 1/10 of 9″ pie   55
  pumpkin *(Sara Lee Homestyle)*, 1/10 of 9″ pie   40

Pie, snack, 1 piece or serving:
  all varieties:
    (Drake's)   0
    (Little Debbie) . . . .   <1
    except lemon *(Hostess)*   15
    lemon *(Hostess)*   30
  frozen, Mississippi mud *(Pepperidge Farm)*   60

Pie crust shell (see also "Pastry shell"):
  frozen, all sizes *(Mrs. Smith's)*, 1/8 shell   0
  frozen, regular, deep dish, or graham cracker *(Pet-Ritz)*, 1/6 shell   7
  frozen, vegetable shortening, all sizes *(Pet Ritz)*, 1/6 shell   0
  mix* *(Flako)*, 1 serving   9
  refrigerator *(Pillsbury* All Ready), 1/8 of 2-crust pie   15

Pie filling, canned, 3.5 oz., except as noted:
  all varieties *(Comstock/Comstock Lite)*, 3.5 oz. . . .   0
  all varieties *(White House)*, 3.5 oz.   0

Pie filling mix, see "Pudding mix"

Pie mix*:
all varieties *(Jell-O No Bake)*, 1/8 pie 30

Pigeon, see "Squab"

Pigeon peas:
fresh or mature, plain 0

Pig's feet:
simmered, 4 oz. 113
pickled, cured, 1 oz. 26

Pike, meat only:
northern:
   raw, 1 lb. 177
   raw, 1 oz. 11
   baked, broiled, or microwaved, 4 oz. 57
walleye, raw, 1 lb. 390
walleye, raw, 1 oz. 24

Pili nuts:
all varieties 0

Pimiento:
all varieties (all brands) 0

Piña colada cocktail mix:
bottled or instant *(Holland House)* 0

Pine nuts:
pignolia or piñon 0

Pineapple:
fresh, canned, or frozen 0

Pineapple juice or drink:
all varieties and blends (all brands) 0

The Cholesterol Content of Food

Pineapple topping:
(Kraft) 0
(Smucker's) 0

Pink beans:
cooked or canned 0

Pinto beans:
cooked, canned, or frozen, w/out sauce 0

Pistachio nuts:
all varieties 0

Pitanga:
fresh 0

Pizza, frozen, 1/4 pie, except as noted:
Canadian bacon *(Totino's Party),* 1/2 pie 10
Canadian-style bacon *(Tombstone)* 40
(Celeste Suprema) 15
(Celeste Suprema Pizza For One), 1 pie 20
cheese:
    (Celeste) 20
    (Celeste Pizza For One), 1 pie 40
    (Tombstone) 30
    (Totino's Microwave), 1 pie 15
    (Totino's Party), 1/2 pie 15
    (Totino's Party Family Size), 1/3 pie 20
    (Weight Watchers), 5.86 oz. 35
cheese, double:
    and hamburger *(Tombstone* Double Top) 75
    and sausage *(Tombstone* Double Top) 80
    and sausage *(Tombstone* Double Top Deluxe) . . 80
cheese, three *(Tombstone* Double Top) 65
cheese, three *(Tombstone* Microwave), 7.7 oz. . . . 60
cheese, two *(Tombstone* Thin Crust) 35
cheese and hamburger *(Tombstone)* 40
cheese and hamburger *(Tombstone* Thin Crust) . . . 40

Pizza *(cont.)*

cheese and pepperoni:

    (Tombstone)   30

    (Tombstone Microwave), 7.5 oz.   50

    (Tombstone Thin Crust)   30

cheese and sausage *(Tombstone)*   40

cheese and sausage *(Tombstone* Thin Crust)   40

cheese, sausage, and mushroom *(Tombstone)* . . .   40

combination:

    (Totino's Microwave), 1 pie   15

    (Totino's Party), 1/2 pie   15

    (Totino's Party Family Size), 1/3 pie   20

    deluxe *(Weight Watchers)*, 7.15 oz.   25

deluxe *(Celeste)*   20

deluxe *(Celeste* Pizza For One), 1 pie   20

hamburger *(Totino's Party)*, 1/2 pie   15

pepperoni:

    (Celeste)   15

    (Celeste Pizza For One), 1 pie   20

    (Tombstone Real Deluxe)   30

    (Totino's Microwave), 1 pie   15

    (Totino's Party), 1/2 pie   20

    (Totino's Party Family Size), 1/3 pie   20

    (Weight Watchers), 6.09 oz.   35

    double cheese *(Tombstone* Double Top)   60

    double cheese *(Tombstone* Double Top Deluxe)   55

sausage:

    (Celeste)   15

    (Celeste Pizza For One), 1 pie   20

    (Tombstone Deluxe)   40

    (Tombstone Deluxe Microwave), 1 pkg.   65

    (Totino's Microwave), 1 pie   10

    (Totino's Party), 1/2 pie   15

    (Totino's Party Family Size), 1/3 pie   20

    (Weight Watchers), 6.26 oz.   35

    Italian *(Tombstone* Microwave), 8 oz.   65

    smoked, w/pepperoni seasoning *(Tombstone)* . .   40

sausage combination *(Tombstone)*   45

sausage and mushroom *(Celeste* Pizza For One),
  1 pie 20
sausage and pepperoni *(Tombstone* Double Top) . . 70
sausage and pepperoni *(Tombstone* Microwave),
  8-oz. pkg. 65

Pizza, French bread, frozen:
  cheese *(Banquet Zap),* 4.5 oz. 35
  deluxe *(Banquet Zap),* 4.8 oz. 25
  deluxe *(Weight Watchers),* 6.12 oz. 30
  pepperoni *(Banquet Zap),* 4.5 oz. 40
  pepperoni *(Weight Watchers),* 5.25 oz. 30

Pizza crust:
  (Pillsbury All Ready), 1/8 crust 0

Pizza dinner, frozen:
  (Kid Cuisine), 6.5 oz. 20

Pizza Hut:
  hand-tossed, medium pie, 2 slices:
    cheese 55
    pepperoni 50
    supreme 55
    super supreme 56
  pan pizza, medium pie, 2 slices:
    cheese 34
    pepperoni 42
    supreme 48
    super supreme 55
  Personal Pan Pizza:
    pepperoni, 1 pie 53
    supreme, 1 pie 49
  Thin 'n Crispy, medium pie, 2 slices:
    cheese 33
    pepperoni 46
    supreme 42
    super supreme 56

Pizza pocket sandwich, frozen:
pepperoni *(Hot Pockets),* 5 oz. 45
sausage *(Hot Pockets),* 5 oz. 65

Pizza sauce:
(Enrico's Homemade Style), 4 oz. 0
(Ragu Pizza Quick), 3 tbsp. 0

Plantain, see "Banana"

Plum:
all varieties, fresh or canned 0

Plum sauce:
tangy *(La Choy)* 0

Poi:
prepared, w/out sauce 0

Pokeberry shoots:
raw or boiled 0

Polish sausage (see also "Kielbasa"):
(Pilgrim's Pride), 3 oz. 72
smoked *(Eckrich Lite* Sausage Links), 1 link 60

Pollack, meat only:
Atlantic, raw, 1 lb. 320
Atlantic, raw, 1 oz. 20
walleye:
raw, 1 lb. 323
raw, 1 oz. 20
baked, broiled, or microwaved, 4 oz. 109

Pomegranate:
fresh 0

Pompano, Florida, meat only:
raw, 1 lb. 227

The Cholesterol Content of Food

raw, 1 oz.	14
baked, broiled, or microwaved, 4 oz.	73

Ponderosa, 1 serving:
chicken, breast	54
chicken wings	75

fish:
bake 'r broil	50
fried	15
nuggets, 1 piece	8
roughy, broiled	28
salmon, broiled	60
scrod, baked	65
shrimp, fried, 7 pieces	105
shrimp, mini, 6 pieces	11
swordfish, broiled	85
trout, broiled	110
hot dog	27

steak:
Kansas City Strip, 5 oz.	76
New York Strip, choice, 8 oz.	50
New York Strip, choice, 10 oz.	62
porterhouse, choice, 16 oz.	82
ribeye, 5 oz.	75
ribeye, choice, 6 oz.	60
sirloin, 7 oz.	63
sirloin tips, 5 oz.	72
steak, chopped, 4 oz.	80
steak kabobs, meat only, 3 oz.	67
steak sandwich, 4 oz.	62
steak teriyaki, 5 oz.	64
T-bone, 8 oz.	71
T-bone, choice, 10 oz.	80

side dishes:
all vegetables, w/out sauce	0
beans, baked	0
cauliflower, okra, or zucchini, breaded, 4 oz.	1
macaroni and cheese, 1 oz.	1

Ponderosa, side dishes (cont.)
onion rings, breaded, 4 oz. 2
potato, baked, 7.2 oz. 0
potato, french fried, 3 oz. 3
potato, mashed, 4 oz. 20
rice pilaf or stuffing, 4 oz. 22
shells, pasta, 2 oz. 0
winter mix, 3.5 oz. 0
salad bar:
chicken salad, 3.5 oz. 42
macaroni salad, 3.5 oz. 9
pasta salad, 3.5 oz. . . . . tr.
potato salad, 3.5 oz. 7
roll, dinner or sourdough 0
turkey ham salad, 3.5 oz. 12
sauce, BBQ or sweet and sour 0
desserts:
banana pudding, 1 oz. 0
ice milk, chocolate, 3.5 oz. 22
ice milk, vanilla, 3.5 oz. 20
mousse, chocolate or strawberry 0
wafer, vanilla, 2 cookies 5

Popcorn, popped (see also "Candy"):
plain (all brands) 0
butter flavor:
(Jiffy Pop) 0
(Jolly Time) 0
(Orville Redenbacher/Orville Redenbacher Lite) . . 0
(Planters) 0
cheddar (Jolly Time) 0
cheddar (Orville Redenbacher), 3 cups 2
cheese flavor (Frito-Lay's) 0
honey caramel (Keebler Pop Deluxe) 0
frozen (Pillsbury Original) 0

Popcorn seasoning:
(McCormick/Schilling Parsley Patch) 0

Poppy seeds:
  (all brands) 0

Pork, fresh, meat only:
  leg, see "Ham"
  loin, whole, lean w/fat:
    braised, 4 oz. 116
    broiled, 4 oz. 107
    broiled, 2.9 oz. (3.7 oz. raw chop w/bone) 77
    roasted, 4 oz. 102
    roasted, diced, 1 cup 126
  loin, whole, lean only:
    braised, 4 oz. 119
    broiled, 4 oz. 108
    broiled, 2.3 oz. (3.7 oz. raw chop w/bone and
      fat) 63
    roasted, 4 oz. 102
    roasted, diced, 1 cup 126
  loin, blade, lean w/fat:
    braised, 4 oz. 122
    broiled, 4 oz. 111
    roasted, 4 oz. 102
  loin, blade, lean only:
    braised, 4 oz. 128
    broiled, 4 oz. 113
    roasted, 4 oz. 101
  loin, center, lean w/fat:
    braised, 4 oz. 121
    broiled, 4 oz. 110
    broiled, 3.1 oz. (3.7 oz. raw chop w/bone) 84
    fried in vegetable oil, 3.1 oz. (4 oz. raw chop
      w/bone) 92
    roasted, 4 oz. 103
  loin, center, lean only:
    braised, 4 oz. 126
    broiled, 4 oz. 111
    broiled, 2.5 oz. (3.7 oz. raw chop w/bone and
      fat) 71

Pork, loin, center, lean only *(cont.)*

    fried in vegetable oil, 2.4 oz. (4 oz. raw chop
        w/bone and fat) 71
    roasted, 4 oz. 103

  loin, center rib, lean w/fat:
    braised, 4 oz. 108
    broiled, 4 oz. 106
    broiled, 2.7 oz. (3.7 oz. raw chop w/bone) 72
    roasted, 4 oz. 92

  loin, center rib, lean only:
    braised, 4 oz. 110
    broiled, 4 oz. 107
    broiled, 2.2 oz. (3.7 oz. raw chop w/bone and
        fat) 59
    roasted, 4 oz. 86

  loin, top, lean w/fat:
    braised, 4 oz. 108
    broiled, 4 oz. 105
    broiled, 3 oz. (3.7 oz. raw chop w/bone) 76

  loin, top, lean only:
    braised, 4 oz. 110
    broiled, 4 oz. 107
    broiled, 2.3 oz. (3.7 oz. raw chop w/bone and
        fat) 60
    roasted, 4 oz. 90

  shoulder, whole, roasted:
    lean w/fat, 4 oz. 109
    lean only, 4 oz. 110

  shoulder, arm (picnic), roasted:
    lean w/fat, 4 oz. 107
    lean w/fat, diced, 1 cup 132
    lean only, 4 oz. 108
    lean only, diced, 1 cup 133

  shoulder, Boston blade, 4 oz.:
    braised, lean w/fat 126
    braised, lean only 132
    broiled, lean w/fat 117
    broiled, lean only 119

roasted, lean only 111
sirloin, lean w/fat:
  braised, 4 oz. 120
  broiled, 4 oz. 110
  broiled, 3 oz. (3.7 oz. raw chop w/bone) 81
  roasted, 4 oz. 103
sirloin, lean only:
  braised, 4 oz. 125
  broiled, 4 oz. 111
  broiled, 2.4 oz. (3.7 oz. raw chop w/bone and
    fat) 67
  roasted, 4 oz. 102
spareribs, lean w/fat, braised, 6.3 oz. (1 lb. raw
  w/bone) 214
tenderloin, roasted:
  lean only, 4 oz. 105
  lean only, diced, 1 cup 130

Pork, cured (see also "Ham"), roasted:
arm (picnic), lean w/fat, 4 oz. 66
arm (picnic), lean only, 4 oz. 54
blade roll, lean w/fat, 4 oz. 76

Pork belly:
raw, 1 oz. 20

Pork entrée, canned:
chow mein (La Choy Bi-Pack), 3/4 cup 14

Pork entrée, frozen or refrigerated, barbecued:
back ribs (John Morrell Pork Classics), 4³/4 oz. . . . 62
chops (John Morrell Pork Classics), 4¹/2 oz. 90
loin (John Morrell Pork Classics), 3 oz. 52
spareribs (John Morrell Pork Classics), 4¹/2 oz. . . . 51
tenderloin (John Morrell Pork Classics), 3 oz. 53

Pork fat:
roasted, 1 oz. 24

Pork rind snack:
(Baken-ets), 1 oz. 25

Pork seasoning and coating mix:
all varieties *(Shake'n Bake)* 0
chop *(McCormick/Schilling* Bag'n Season) 0

Pork and beans, see "Baked beans"

Pot roast, see "Beef dinner" and "Beef entrée, frozen"

Pot roast seasoning mix:
(Lawry's Seasoning Blends) 0
(McCormick/Schilling Bag'n Season) 0

Potato (see also "Potato dishes"):
fresh, canned, dried, or frozen, w/out sauce 0
frozen, fried or french-fried:
  plain, all cuts *(Heinz Deep Fries)* 0
  plain, all cuts *(Ore-Ida)* 0
  w/onions *(Ore-Ida Crispy Crowns)* 0
frozen, hash brown:
  all varieties, except cheddar *(Ore-Ida)* 0
  w/butter and onions *(Heinz Deep Fries)*, 3 oz. ... 5
  w/cheddar *(Ore-Ida Cheddar Browns)*, 3 oz. 10
frozen, O'Brien *(Ore-Ida)* 0
frozen, puffs, all varieties *(Ore-Ida Tater Tots)* 0

Potato, stuffed, see "Potato dishes, frozen"

Potato, sweet, see "Sweet potato"

Potato chips and crisps, 1 oz.:
(Munchos) 0
all varieties, all flavors *(Bachman)* 0
all varieties, all flavors *(Cape Cod)* 0
all varieties, all flavors *(Eagle)* 0
all varieties, all flavors *(Lay's)* 0

The Cholesterol Content of Food

all varieties, all flavors *(O'Boisies)* 0
all varieties, all flavors *(Ruffles)* 0
skins, all varieties, all flavors *(Tato Skins)* 0

Potato dishes, canned or packaged:
au gratin *(Green Giant Pantry Express)*, 1/2 cup . . . 5
scalloped, and ham *(Hormel Micro-Cup)*, 7.5 oz. . . . 25

Potato dishes, frozen:
au gratin *(Birds Eye For One)*, 5.5 oz. 30
au gratin *(Green Giant* One Serving), 5.5 oz. 20
and broccoli, w/cheese sauce *(Green Giant* One
    Serving), 5.5 oz. 5
cheddared *(The Budget Gourmet)*, 5.5 oz. 35
cheddared, and broccoli *(The Budget Gourmet)*,
    5 oz. 25
nacho *(The Budget Gourmet)*, 5 oz. 30
new, in sour cream sauce *(The Budget Gourmet)*,
    5 oz. 20
shredded, w/vegetables, in cheese sauce *(Stokely
    Singles)*, 4.5 oz. 15
sliced, w/bacon, in cheddar cheese sauce *(Stokely
    Singles)*, 4.5 oz. 10
stuffed, 6 oz.:
    w/bacon *(Oh Boy!)* 5
    w/cheddar *(Oh Boy!)* 6
    w/sour cream & chives *(Oh Boy!)* 2
stuffed, baked:
    broccoli and cheese *(Weight Watchers)*, 10.5 oz. 25
    chicken divan *(Weight Watchers)*, 11 oz. 40
    ham Lorraine *(Weight Watchers)*, 11 oz. 15
    turkey, homestyle *(Weight Watchers)*, 12 oz. . . . 60
three cheese *(The Budget Gourmet* Side Dish),
    5.75 oz. 30

Potato dishes, mix*, 1/2 cup:
au gratin *(Kraft* Potatoes & Cheese) 40
broccoli au gratin *(Kraft* Potatoes & Cheese) 40
scalloped *(Kraft* Potatoes & Cheese) 25

Potato dishes, mix* *(cont.)*
   scalloped, w/ham *(Kraft* Potatoes & Cheese)   15
   sour cream w/chives *(Kraft* Potatoes & Cheese) . .   10
   two cheese *(Kraft* Potatoes & Cheese)   10

Potato flour or starch:
   plain or blend   0

Potato salad seasoning:
   (Tone's)   0

Poultry, see specific listings

Poultry seasoning:
   (all brands)   0

Pout, ocean, meat only:
   raw, 1 lb.   236
   raw, 1 oz.   15

Praline pecan mousse, frozen:
   (Weight Watchers), 2.71 oz.   5

Preserves:
   all varieties (all brands)   0

Pretzel:
   (A & Eagle)   0
   all varieties *(Bachman)*   0
   all varieties *(Quinlan)*   0
   all varieties *(Rold Gold)*   0
   braids or knots *(Keebler* Butter)   0

Prickly pear:
   fresh   0

Prune:
   canned, dehydrated, or dried   0

The Cholesterol Content of Food

Prune juice:
(all brands) 0

Pudding, ready-to-serve:
all flavors:
   (Hunt's Snack Pack) 0
   (Hunt's Snack Pack Lite) 0
   (Jell-O Light Pudding Snacks), 4 oz. 5
   (Jell-O Pudding Snacks) 0
   (Swiss Miss), 4 oz. 1
   (Swiss Miss Lite) 0
   except tapioca *(Crowley)*, 4.5 oz. 10
tapioca *(Crowley)*, 4.5 oz. 5

Pudding, frozen:
all flavors *(Rich's)* 0

Pudding bar, frozen:
all flavors *(Jell-O Pudding Pops)* 0

Pudding mix*, 1/2 cup:
all flavors:
   (Salada Danish Dessert) 0
   w/whole milk *(Jell-O/Jell-O Instant/Microwave)* . . 15
   w/2% lowfat milk *(Jell-O Instant Sugar Free)* . . . 10
   w/skim milk *(D-Zerta)* 0
   custard, egg, golden *(Jell-O Americana)* 80
   rice or vanilla tapioca *(Jell-O Americana)* 15

Pummelo:
fresh 0

Pumpkin:
fresh or canned 0

Pumpkin leaf or flower:
raw or cooked 0

Pumpkin pie spice:
  (all brands)   0

Pumpkin seeds:
  roasted or dried   0

Purslane:
  raw or boiled   0

Q

Food and Measure	Cholesterol (mgs.)
Quince:	
fresh	0
Quinoa:	
1 oz.	0

R

Food and Measure	Cholesterol (mgs.)
Rabbit, meat only:	
domesticated:	
roasted, 4 oz.	73
stewed, 4 oz.	98
stewed, diced, 1 cup	120
wild, stewed, 4 oz.	139
wild, stewed, diced, 1 cup	172
Radish:	
all varieties, fresh	0
Raisins:	
all varieties (all brands)	0

Raspberry:
fresh or frozen   0

Raspberry danish, frozen:
twist *(Sara Lee),* 1/8 pkg.   15

Raspberry drink or juice:
all blends (all brands)   0

Ravioli, canned or packaged, 7.5 oz.:
beef *(Chef Boyardee* Microwave)   11
beef, in tomato sauce *(Hormel Micro-Cup)*   21
cheese, in meat sauce *(Chef Boyardee* Microwave)   10
cheese or meat, in sauce *(Buitoni)*   5

Ravioli, frozen:
cheese *(Buitoni),* 4 oz.   65

Ravioli entrée, frozen:
cheese *(The Budget Gourmet Slim Selects),* 10 oz.   45
cheese, baked *(Weight Watchers),* 9 oz.   85

Rax, 1 serving:
sandwiches:
   BBC   137
   BBQ   24
   fish . . . .   <1
   ham and Swiss   37
   Philly beef, w/cheese   49
   roast beef   36
   roast beef, large   36
   roast beef, small (Uncle Al)   19
   turkey bacon club   87
french fries, large   16
french fries, regular   10
potatoes:
   plain, w/margarine   0
   BBQ, w/cheese   18
   cheese and bacon   23

Rax, potatoes *(cont.)*

cheese and broccoli	11
chili and cheese	25
Mexican bar:	
cheese sauce, plain or nacho, 3.5 oz.	11
refried beans, 3 oz.	2
sour topping, 3.5 oz.	<1
Spanish rice, 3.5 oz.	0
spicy meat sauce, 3.5 oz.	12
taco sauce or shells	0
tortilla or tortilla chips	0
pasta bar, 3.5 oz.:	
Alfredo sauce	10
pasta shells	0
pasta/vegetable blend	0
rainbow rotini	2
spaghetti	0
spaghetti sauce, plain or w/meat	<1
chocolate chip cookie, 1 piece	<1
milkshake, w/out whipped topping:	
chocolate	63
strawberry	62
vanilla	58
whipped topping, 1 dollop	2

Red beans:

cooked or canned	0

Red snapper, see "Snapper"

Redfish, see "Ocean perch"

Refried beans, canned:

plain or spicy *(Old El Paso)*, 1/4 cup	1
w/cheese *(Old El Paso)*, 1/4 cup	2
vegetarian *(Old El Paso)*, 1/4 cup	0

The Cholesterol Content of Food

Relish:
    all varieties *(Heinz)*   0
    all varieties *(Vlasic)*   0
    pickle *(Claussen)*   0

Rhubarb:
    fresh or frozen   0

Rib sauce:
    (Dip n'Joy Saucey Rib)   0

Rice (see also "Rice dishes"):
    all varieties, cooked w/out butter, broth, or sauce
        (all brands)   0

Rice, wild, see "Wild rice"

Rice bran:
    crude or processed   0

Rice cake:
    all varieties *(Quaker)*   0
    all varieties, except cheese *(Hain Mini)*, 1/2 oz. . . .   0
    cheese, regular or nacho *(Hain Mini)*, 1/2 oz. . . . . .   <5

Rice dishes, canned:
    fried *(La Choy)*, 3/4 cup   0
    Spanish *(Old El Paso)*, 1/2 cup   0

Rice dishes, frozen:
    (Green Giant Rice Originals Medley), 1/2 cup   5
    and broccoli, au gratin *(Birds Eye For One)*,
        5.75 oz.   5
    and broccoli, in cheese sauce *(Green Giant* One
        Serving), 5.5 oz.   5
    French style *(Birds Eye)*, 3.3 oz.   0
    Italian, w/spinach, in cheese sauce *(Green Giant*
        Rice Originals), 1/2 cup   10

Rice dishes, frozen *(cont.)*
  Oriental, and vegetables *(The Budget Gourmet
    Side Dish)*, 5.75 oz.   20
  peas and mushrooms, w/sauce *(Green Giant One
    Serving)*, 5.5 oz.   5
  pilaf *(Green Giant Rice Originals)*, 1/2 cup   2
  pilaf, w/green beans *(The Budget Gourmet Side
    Dish)*, 5.5 oz.   10
  Spanish style *(Birds Eye)*, 3.3 oz.   0
  white and wild *(Green Giant Rice Originals)*, 1/2 cup   0
  wild, sherry *(Green Giant* Microwave Garden
    Gourmet)*, 1 pkg.   10

Rice dishes, mix*, 1/2 cup, except as noted:
  all varieties *(Minute Microwave Family Size)*   10
  all varieties, except fried *(Minute)*   10
  all varieties, except cheddar and broccoli *(Minute
    Microwave Single Size)*   5
  almondine *(Hain 3-Grain Side Dish)*   0
  au gratin, herb *(Success)*   0
  cheddar and broccoli *(Minute* Microwave Single
    Size)   10
  fried *(Minute)*   0
  Mexican *(Old El Paso)*   0

Rice flour:
  brown or white   0

Rigatoni entrée, canned:
  (Chef Boyardee Microwave)*, 7.5 oz.   17

Rigatoni entrée, frozen:
  bake, w/meat sauce and cheese *(Lean Cuisine)*,
    9.75 oz.   40

"Roast," vegetarian, frozen:
  (Worthington Dinner Roast)   0

The Cholesterol Content of Food

Robert sauce:
  (Escoffier) 0

Rockfish, meat only:
  raw, 1 lb. 156
  raw, 1 oz. 10
  baked, broiled, or microwaved, 4 oz. 50

Roe (see also "Caviar"):
  1 oz. 106
  1 tbsp. 60

Roll, 1 piece, except as noted:
  assorted *(Brownberry* Hearth) 7
  brown and serve, all varieties *(du Jour)* 0
  brown and serve, all varieties *(Pepperidge Farm)* . . 0
  crescent, butter *(Pepperidge Farm)* 15
  croissant, see "Croissant"
  dinner:
    (Arnold 24 Dinner Party) 1
    (Pepperidge Farm Country Style/Party/Soft) 0
    (Roman Meal Original) 0
    all varieties *(Awrey's)* 0
    old-fashioned or Parkerhouse *(Pepperidge Farm)* 5
    poppy seed, finger *(Pepperidge Farm)* . . . . <5
    potato classic, hearty *(Pepperidge Farm)* 0
    wheat or white *(Home Pride)* 0
  egg *(Levy's* Old Country Deli), 1 oz. 11
  egg sandwich *(Arnold* Dutch) 1
  French style *(Francisco* International) 0
  French style, all varieties *(Pepperidge Farm)* 0
  hamburger or hot dog:
    (Arnold) 0
    (Pepperidge Farm) 0
    (Roman Meal Original) 0
  hoagie *(Pepperidge Farm* Soft) 0
  kaiser *(Arnold* Francisco) 5
  kaiser *(Brownberry* Hearth) 9
  onion *(Levy's* Old Country Deli), 1 oz. 11

Roll *(cont.)*
  sandwich:
    all varieties, except salad *(Pepperidge Farm)*   0
    oat bran *(Awrey's)*   0
    salad *(Pepperidge Farm)*   10
  steak, sweet *(Colombo* Brand)   0
  twist, golden *(Pepperidge Farm)*   5
  frozen, Parkerhouse *(Bridgford)*   0
  refrigerated, all varieties *(Pillsbury)*   0

Roll, sweet (see also "Bun, sweet"), 1 piece:
  cinnamon:
    (Hostess Breakfast Bake Shop)   20
    homestyle *(Awrey's)*   5
    swirl *(Awrey's* Grande)   10
  orange or pecan-caramel swirl *(Hostess Breakfast
    Bake Shop)*   10
  pecan *(Hostess Breakfast Bake Shop* Spinners) . . .   5
  frozen, apple or cheese *(Weight Watchers)*   5
  frozen, strawberry *(Weight Watchers)*   20
  refrigerated, cinnamon, iced *(Pillsbury)*   0

Roman beans, canned:
  (Progresso)   0

Roseapple:
  fresh   0

Roselle:
  fresh   0

Rosemary:
  fresh or dried (all brands)   0

Rotini entrée, frozen:
  cheddar *(Green Giant* Microwave Garden Gourmet),
    1 pkg.   20
  seafood *(Mrs. Paul's* Light), 9 oz.   25

Roughy, orange, meat only, raw:

1 lb.	91
1 oz.	6

Roy Rogers, 1 serving:

crescent roll	<5
crescent sandwich:	
regular	207
w/bacon	212
w/ham	227
w/sausage	248
egg and biscuit platter:	
regular	417
w/bacon	424
w/ham	437
w/sausage	458
pancake platter, w/syrup and butter:	
regular	51
w/bacon	58
w/ham	71
w/sausage	92
chicken, fried:	
breast	118
breast and wing	165
drumstick	40
drumstick and thigh	125
nuggets, 6 pieces	63
thigh	85
wing	47
sandwiches:	
bacon cheeseburger	83
bar burger	96
cheeseburger	76
cheeseburger, small	36
hamburger	64
hamburger, small	26
*Express*burger	70
Express bacon cheeseburger	89

Roy Rogers, sandwiches *(cont.)*
   Express cheeseburger 82
   fish 62
   roast beef 58
   roast beef, w/cheese 70
   roast beef, large 82
   roast beef, large, w/cheese 94
  side dishes:
   biscuit . . . . <5
   coleslaw . . . . <5
   french fries 13
   french fries, small 10
   french fries, large 19
  shakes:
   chocolate 37
   strawberry 37
   vanilla 40
  sundaes:
   caramel 23
   hot fudge 23
   strawberry 23
  Vitari, 1 oz. 9

Rutabaga:
  fresh or canned, plain 0

Rye (see also "Rye flour"):
  whole-grain 0

Rye cake:
  (Quaker Grain Cakes) 0

Rye flour:
  dark, light, or medium 0
  and wheat *(Pillsbury's Best* Bohemian Style) 0

S

Food and Measure	Cholesterol (mgs.)
Sablefish, meat only:	
raw, 1 lb.	222
raw, 1 oz.	14
smoked, 4 oz.	73
Safflower seed kernels:	
raw or dried	0
Safflower seed meal:	
all varieties	0
Saffron:	
threads or powder	0

Sage:
    fresh or dried (all brands)   0

Salad dip:
    (Nasoya Vegi-Dip)   0

Salad dressing, 1 tbsp., except as noted:
    (Ott's Famous) . . . .   <1
    all varieties:
        (Kraft Free/Kraft Free Catalina)   0
        (Seven Seas Free/Seven Seas Viva Free)   0
        except French mustard *(Hain Canola Oil)*   0
        except Thousand Island *(Hollywood)*   0
        except buttermilk, blue cheese, coleslaw,
          Russian, and Thousand Island *(Kraft)*   0
        except Thousand Island *(Seven Seas Light)*   0
        except ranch *(Seven Seas Viva Light)*   0
    balsamic vinegar and oil *(Great Impressions)*   0
    blue cheese:
        (Roka Brand)   10
        (Roka Brand Reduced Calorie) . . . .   <5
        chunky *(Kraft/Kraft* Reduced Calorie) . . . .   <5
        chunky *(Wish-Bone/Wish-Bone* Lite)   1
    buttermilk:
        (Hain Old Fashioned)   0
        (Seven Seas Buttermilk Recipe)   5
        creamy *(Kraft/Kraft* Reduced Calorie) . . . .   <5
    Caesar *(Wish-Bone)*   1
    Caesar, creamy *(Hain/Hain* Low Salt) . . . .   <5
    Chinese vinegar, w/sesame and ginger *(Lawry's*
      Classic)   0
    coleslaw *(Kraft)*   10
    coleslaw *(Miracle Whip)*   5
    creamy *(Rancher's Choice)*   5
    creamy *(Rancher's Choice* Reduced Calorie)   5
    cucumber dill *(Hain)*   5
    Dijon mustard *(Great Impressions)*   18

The Cholesterol Content of Food

Dijon vinaigrette:
   (Hain) . . . .   <5
   (Wish-Bone Classic) . . . .   <1
   (Wish-Bone Lite Classic)   0
dill, creamy *(Nasoya Vegi-Dressing)*   0
French:
   (Catalina)   0
   all varieties *(Wish-Bone)*   0
   creamy *(Hain)*   0
   creamy *(Seven Seas)*   0
   w/green pepper *(Great Impressions)*   0
French mustard, spicy *(Hain* Canola Oil)   5
garlic:
   creamy or French *(Wish-Bone)*   0
   herb *(Nasoya Vegi-Dressing)*   0
   and sour cream *(Hain)*   0
herb, savory *(Hain* No Salt)   0
herb and spice *(Seven Seas Viva)*   0
honey and sesame *(Hain)*   0
Italian:
   (Nasoya Vegi-Dressing)   0
   (Ott's) . . . .   <1
   (Seven Seas/Seven Seas Viva)   0
   (Wish-Bone/Wish-Bone Blended)   0
   (Wish-Bone Lite/Robusto)   0
   cheese vinaigrette *(Hain)* . . . .   <5
   w/cheese *(Wish-Bone)* . . . .   <1
   creamy or traditional *(Hain/Hain* No Salt)   0
   creamy *(Wish-Bone/Wish-Bone* Lite) . . . .   <1
   herbal *(Wish-Bone* Classics)   0
mayonnaise, see "Mayonnaise"
mayonnaise type:
   (Kraft Free)   0
   (Miracle Whip)   5
   (Miracle Whip Free/Miracle Whip Light)   0
   (Spin Blend)   10
   cholesterol free *(Spin Blend)*   0

Salad dressing *(cont.)*
  olive oil:
    Italian *(Wish-Bone Classic)*   0
    vinaigrette *(Wish-Bone/Wish-Bone Lite)*   0
  onion and chive *(Wish-Bone Lite)*   0
  poppyseed *(Hain Rancher's)* . . . .   <5
  ranch:
    (Seven Seas Viva/Seven Seas Viva Light)   5
    (Wish-Bone)   4
    (Wish-Bone Lite)   5
    creamy *(Weight Watchers)*   0
  red wine vinaigrette *(Wish-Bone)*   0
  red wine vinegar and oil *(Great Impressions)*   0
  red wine vinegar and oil *(Seven Seas Viva)*   0
  Russian *(Wish-Bone/Wish-Bone Lite)*   0
  Russian, creamy *(Kraft)*   5
  sesame garlic *(Nasoya Vegi-Dressing)*   0
  sesame seed   0
  sour *(Friendship Sour Treat)*   0
  Swiss cheese vinaigrette *(Hain)* . . . .   <5
  Thousand Island:
    (Hain)   0
    (Hollywood)   5
    (Kraft/Kraft Reduced Calorie)   5
    (Seven Seas Light)   5
    (Wish-Bone)   7
    (Wish-Bone Lite)   9
    and bacon *(Kraft)*   0
    creamy *(Seven Seas)*   5
  white wine vinegar and oil *(Great Impressions)* . . .   0

Salad dressing mix*, 1 tbsp.:
  all varieties, except buttermilk and ranch *(Good
    Seasons/Good Seasons Lite)*   0
  all varieties, except bleu cheese and Thousand
    Island *(Hain No Oil)*   0
  bleu cheese *(Hain No Oil)* . . . .   <5
  buttermilk *(Good Seasons Farm Style)*   5

ranch *(Good Seasons/Good Seasons Lite)* 5
Thousand Island *(Hain No Oil)* . . . . <1

Salad seasoning:
(McCormick/Shilling Salad Supreme) 0

Salami:
beef:
   (Boar's Head), 1 oz. 20
   (Hebrew National), 1 oz. 15
   (Oscar Mayer Machiaeh Brand), .8-oz. slice 15
beer *(Oscar Mayer* Salami for Beer), .8-oz. slice . . 15
beer, beef *(Oscar Mayer* Salami for Beer), .8-oz.
   slice 16
cotto:
   regular or beef *(Oscar Mayer),* .5-oz. slice 12
   regular or beef *(Oscar Mayer),* .8-oz. slice 19
dry or hard *(Oscar Mayer* Hard), .3-oz. slice 8
Genoa *(Oscar Mayer),* .3-oz. slice 9

"Salami," vegetarian, frozen:
roll or slices *(Worthington)* 0

Salisbury steak, see "Beef dinner" and "Beef
entrée"

Salmon, fresh, meat only:
Atlantic, raw, 1 lb. 249
Atlantic, raw, 1 oz. 16
Chinook:
   raw, 1 lb. 299
   raw, 1 oz. 19
   lox, 4 oz. 26
   smoked, 4 oz. 26
chum, raw, 1 lb. 336
chum, raw, 1 oz. 21
Coho:
   raw, 1 lb. 177

Salmon, Coho *(cont.)*

raw, 1 oz.	11
boiled, poached, or steamed, 4 oz.	56
pink, raw, 1 lb.	236
pink, raw, 1 oz.	15
sockeye:	
raw, 1 lb.	283
raw, 1 oz.	18
baked, broiled, or microwaved, 4 oz.	99

Salmon, canned:

chum, drained, 4 oz.	44
pink or red sockeye, Alaska *(Deming's)*, 1/2 cup	65

Salmon, frozen:

steaks, w/out seasoning *(SeaPak)*, 8-oz. pkg.	170

Salsa:

all varieties *(Del Monte)*	0
all varieties *(Hain)*	0
all varieties *(La Victoria)*	0
all varieties *(Old El Paso)*	0
all varieties *(Ortega)*	0
mild or hot *(Enrico's* Chunky)	0
taco, mild *(Rosarita)*, 2 oz.	<1
Texas *(Hot Cha Cha)*	0

Salsify:

all varieties, raw or boiled	0

Salt:

all varieties	0

Salt, substitute:

(all brands)	0

Salt pork:

raw, 1 oz.	25

The Cholesterol Content of Food

Sandwich, see specific listings

Sandwich spread:
(Hellmann's/Best Foods), 1 tbsp.   5
(Kraft), 1 tbsp.   5
meat *(Oscar Mayer Chub)*, 1 oz.   10

Sapodilla:
fresh   0

Sapote:
fresh   0

Sardine, fresh, see "Herring"

Sardine, canned:
Atlantic, in oil, drained:
2 oz.   81
2 medium, 3" × 1" × 1/2"   34

Pacific, in tomato sauce, drained:
2 oz.   35
1 medium, 4³/4" × 1¹/8" × ⁵/8"   23

Sauce, see specific listings

Sauerkraut:
canned or chilled (all brands)   0

Sauerkraut juice:
(all brands)   0

Sausage (see also specific listings), 1 link or patty,
except as noted:
beef *(Jones Dairy Farm* Golden Brown)   18
brown and serve *(Jones Dairy Farm* Light)   16
Italian, see "Italian sausage"
pork:
(Jones Dairy Farm)   24
(Jones Dairy Farm Golden Brown Light)   16

Sausage, pork *(cont.)*
    (Jones Dairy Farm Light) 21
    cooked *(Oscar Mayer Little Friers)* 17
    fresh, cooked, .5 oz. (1 oz. raw link) 11
    mild or spicy *(Jones Dairy Farm* Golden Brown) 18
  pork, patty:
    fresh, cooked, 1 oz. (2 oz. raw patty) 22
    (Jones Dairy Farm) 36
    (Jones Dairy Farm Golden Brown) 29
  pork roll *(Jones Dairy Farm* Cello Roll), 1 slice . . . 24
  smoked:
    (Eckrich Lite) 35
    (Eckrich Lite Sausage Links) 60
    (Eckrich Lite Smok-Y-Links), 2 links 25
    (Oscar Mayer Little Smokies) 6
    (Oscar Mayer Smokie Links) 28
    (Pilgrim's Pride), 3 oz. 64
    beef *(Eckrich Lite* Sausage Links) 60
    beef *(Oscar Mayer* Smokies) 27
    cheddar *(Eckrich Lite* Sausage Links) 70
    cheese *(Oscar Mayer* Smokies) 28
  sticks, see "Beef jerky"

"Sausage," vegetarian:
  canned or frozen, all varieties *(Worthington)* 0
  frozen, all varieties *(Morningstar Farms)* 0

Sausage breakfast biscuit, frozen:
  (Weight Watchers), 3 oz. 70

Sausage breakfast taco:
  (Owens Border Breakfasts), 2.17 oz. 65

Sausage seasoning:
  pork *(Tone's)* 0

Savory:
  fresh or dried 0

The Cholesterol Content of Food

Scallion, see "Onion, green"

Scallop:
fresh, meat only, raw, 1 lb. 152
fresh, meat only, raw, 2 large or 5 small 10
frozen, fried *(Mrs. Paul's),* 3 oz. 10

Scallop, imitation (from surimi):
1 lb. 98
1 oz. 6

"Scallop," vegetarian, canned:
(Worthington Vegetable Skallops) 0

Scallop and shrimp dinner, frozen:
Mariner *(The Budget Gourmet),* 11.5 oz. 70

Scallop squash:
fresh or frozen 0

Scrapple:
(Jones Dairy Farm), 1 slice 24

Scrod, fresh, see "Cod, Atlantic"

Scrod entrée, frozen:
baked *(Gorton's Microwave Entrees),* 1 pkg. 80

Sea bass (see also "Bass"), meat only:
raw, 1 lb. 186
raw, 1 oz. 12
baked, broiled, or microwaved, 4 oz. 60

Seafood, see specific listings

Seafood dinner, frozen:
w/herbs *(Armour Classics Lite),* 10 oz. 35

Seafood entrée, frozen:
combination platter, breaded *(Mrs. Paul's),* 9 oz. . . . 85
Newberg *(The Budget Gourmet),* 10 oz. 70
Newberg *(Healthy Choice),* 8 oz. 55

Seafood sauce (see also "Cocktail sauce"):
(Progresso Authentic Pasta Sauces), 1/2 cup 95
mixed *(Progresso),* 1/2 cup 11

Seafood and crabmeat salad:
(Longacre Saladfest), 1 oz. 5

Seasoned coating mix, see specific listings

Sea trout (see also "Trout"), meat only:
raw, 1 lb. 376
raw, 1 oz. 24

Seaweed:
all varieties, fresh or dried 0

Semolina:
whole-grain or flour 0

Sesame butter, see "Sesame paste" and "Tahini"

Sesame chips:
(Flavor Tree) 0

Sesame flour or meal:
all varieties 0

Sesame nut mix:
dry-roasted *(Planters)* 0

Sesame paste (see also "Tahini"):
plain, all varieties 0

Sesame seasoning:
  all-purpose *(McCormick/Schilling Parsley Patch)* . .   0

Sesame seeds:
  all varieties   0

Sesame sticks:
  (Flavor Tree)   0

Sesbania flower:
  raw or steamed   0

7-Eleven, 1 serving:
  Big Bite   27
  Big Bite Super   54
  burrito:
    bean and cheese   46
    beef, bean, and cheese   40
    beef and potato   32
    chicken and rice   13
  burrito, beef and bean:
    5 oz.   23
    green chili   46
    red chili   23
    red hot, 5 oz.   23
    red hot, 10 oz.   47
    red hot, premium   31
  chicken breast, 4.8 oz.   29
  enchilada, beef and cheese   55
  fajitas   32
  sandito, ham and cheese   40
  sandito, pizza   23
  tacos, soft, twin   50
  Deli-Shoppe microwave products:
    bacon cheeseburger   11
    bagel and cream cheese   47
    char sandwich, large   11

7-Eleven, Deli-Shoppe microwave products *(cont.)*
  fish sandwich, w/cheese 11
  sausage, red hot, large 128
  turkey wedge, 3.4 oz. 24

Shakey's:
  pizza, *Homestyle Pan Crust,* 1/10 of 12" pie:
    cheese 21
    onion, green peppers, olives, mushrooms 21
    pepperoni 27
    sausage, mushroom 24
    sausage, pepperoni 24
    Shakey's Special 29
  pizza, thick crust, 1/10 of 12" pie:
    cheese 13
    green pepper, olives, mushrooms 13
    pepperoni 17
    sausage, mushrooms 15
    sausage, pepperoni 19
    Shakey's Special 18
  pizza, thin crust, 1/10 of 12" pie:
    cheese 14
    onion, green pepper, olives, mushrooms 11
    pepperoni 14
    sausage, mushroom 13
    sausage, pepperoni 17
    Shakey's Special 16

Shallot:
  fresh or freeze-dried 0

Shark, meat only:
  raw, 1 lb. 232
  raw, 1 oz. 14

Shellie beans:
  canned, w/out sauce 0

Shells, stuffed, dinner, frozen:
three cheese (*Le Menu* LightStyle), 10 oz.   25

Shells, stuffed, entrée, frozen:
(*Buitoni* Single Serving), 9 oz.   80
w/vegetables (*Legume* Provencale), 11 oz.   0

Sherbet (see also "Sorbet" and "Ice"):
all flavors (*Sealtest*), 1/2 cup   5

Sherbet bar, frozen, 1 bar:
all flavors (*Fudgsicle* Fat Free)   0
all flavors (*Fudgsicle* Sugar Free)   5

Shoney's:
breakfast (kitchen ordered):
bacon, 3 strips   16
biscuit, 1 piece   0
bun, honey, 1 piece   3
country gravy, 3 oz.   2
croissant, 1 piece   2
egg, fried, 1 egg 274
grits, hash browns, or home fries, 3 oz.   0
ham, breakfast, 2 slices   28
muffin, blueberry, 2 pieces   33
pancake, 6" cake, 2.3 oz.   0
sausage patty, 1 piece   17
sirloin steak, charbroiled, 6 oz.   99
toast, buttered, 2 slices   0
burgers and sandwiches:
All-American burger   86
bacon burger   86
baked ham sandwich   42
charbroiled chicken.   90
chicken fillet sandwich   51
country fried sandwich   29
fish sandwich   21
grilled bacon & cheese sandwich   36
grilled cheese sandwich.   36

Shoney's, burgers and sandwiches *(cont.)*

ham club on whole wheat	78
mushroom/Swiss burger	106
Old-Fashioned burger	82
patty melt	121
Philly steak sandwich	103
Reuben sandwich	138
Shoney burger	79
Slim Jim sandwich	57
turkey club on whole wheat	100

entrées, 1 serving:

beef patty, light	82
chicken tenders	64
fish, baked	83
fish, fried, light	65
Fish N' Chips (includes fries)	103
Fish N' Shrimp	127
Italian Feast	74
lasagna	26
Liver N' Onions	529
seafood platter	127
shrimp, bite-size	140
shrimp, boiled	182
shrimp, charbroiled	162
shrimp sampler	217
Shrimper's Feast	125
Shrimper's Feast, large	188
spaghetti	55
steak, country fried	27

steak and chicken, charbroiled:

chicken	85
chicken, Hawaiian	85
Half O' Pound	123
ribeye, 8 oz.	141
sirloin, 6 oz.	99
Steak N' Shrimp (fried)	150
Steak N' Shrimp (charbroiled)	141

soup, 6 oz.:

bean	4
beef-cabbage	13
broccoli, cream of	1
broccoli-cauliflower	12
cheese Florentine ham	11
chicken, cream of	11
chicken noodle	14
chicken rice	6
clam chowder	0
onion	1
potato	0
tomato Florentine or tomato vegetable	0
vegetable beef	5

side dishes:

baked potato, plain	0
bread, Grecian	0
french fries	0
mushrooms, sauteed, 3 oz.	0
onion rings, 1 ring	2
onions, sauteed	0
rice, 3.5 oz.	1

sauces, 1 soufflé cup:

BBQ, cocktail, or sweet N' sour	0
tartar	11

salad, prepared, 1/4 cup:

ambrosia	0
beet-onion	0
broccoli and cauliflower	0
broccoli and cauliflower, ranch	9
broccoli, cauliflower, carrot	1
carrot apple	8
coleslaw	7
cucumber, lite	0
fruit, mixed or fruit delight	0
Italian vegetable	0
kidney bean	2
macaroni	14

Corinne T. Netzer

Shoney's, salad, prepared, 1/4 cup *(cont.)*

Oriental	1
pasta, rotelli or Don's	0
pea	42
pistachio-pineapple	0
Seigan	5
snow	0
spaghetti	0
spring or summer	0
squash, mixed	0
three bean	0
Waldorf	2

salad dressings, 2 tbsp.:

Biscayne, lo-Cal	0
blue cheese	15
French	12
French, Rue	0
honey mustard	18
Italian, all varieties	0
ranch	15
Thousand Island	12

desserts, 1 serving:

apple pie à la mode	35
carrot cake	37
hot fudge cake	27
hot fudge sundae	60
strawberry pie	0
strawberry sundae	69
walnut brownie à la mode	35

Shortening:

vegetable blends, all varieties	0

Shrimp:

fresh, meat only:

raw, 1 lb.	692
raw, 1 oz. or 4 large	43
boiled or steamed, 4 oz.	221

The Cholesterol Content of Food

```
boiled or steamed, 4 large . . . . . . . . . . . . .      43
canned, drained, 1 cup . . . . . . . . . . . . . . . .   222
```

Shrimp, imitation (from surimi):
```
1 lb. . . . . . . . . . . . . . . . . . . . . . . . .   163
1 oz. . . . . . . . . . . . . . . . . . . . . . . . .    10
```

Shrimp dinner, frozen:
```
baby bay (Armour Classics Lite), 9.75 oz. . . . . . .   105
creole (Armour Classics Lite), 11.25 oz. . . . . . . .   45
creole (Healthy Choice), 11.25 oz. . . . . . . . . . .   65
marinara (Healthy Choice), 10.5 oz. . . . . . . . . .    50
```

Shrimp entrée, canned:
```
chow mein (La Choy Bi-Pack), 3/4 cup . . . . . . . .     19
```

Shrimp entrée, frozen:
```
battered (SeaPak), 4 oz. . . . . . . . . . . . . . . .    20
breaded, butterfly (SeaPak Mikado), 4 oz. . . . . . .   110
breaded, crunchy (Gorton's Microwave), 5 oz. . . .      65
and chicken Cantonese, w/noodles (Lean Cuisine),
  10 1/8 oz. . . . . . . . . . . . . . . . . . . . .    100
and clams, w/linguini (Mrs. Paul's Light), 10 oz. . .    40
and fettucine (The Budget Gourmet), 9.5 oz. . . . .    145
w/lobster sauce (La Choy Fresh & Lite), 10 oz. . . .   118
primavera (Right Course), 9 5/8 oz. . . . . . . . . .    50
```

Shrimp salad:
```
(Longacre Saladfest), 1 oz. . . . . . . . . . . . . .    25
w/seafood (Longacre Saladfest), 1 oz. . . . . . . . .    15
```

Shrimp spice:
```
(Tone's Craboil), 1 tsp. . . . . . . . . . . . . . . .     1
```

Skipper's:
thick-cut cod:
```
3 piece, fries . . . . . . . . . . . . . . . . . . . .    38
4 piece, fries . . . . . . . . . . . . . . . . . . . .    50
5 piece, fries . . . . . . . . . . . . . . . . . . . .    62
```

Skipper's *(cont.)*
famous fish fillets:
  1 fish, fries 55
  2 fish, fries 108
  3 fish, fries 160
seafood combo, w/fries:
  clam strips, 1 fish 61
  oysters, 1 fish 80
  shrimp, 1 fish 105
  jumbo shrimp, 1 fish 91
seafood basket, w/fries:
  clam strips 14
  oysters 52
  shrimp 102
  jumbo shrimp 73
  Skipper's Platter 111
chicken tenderloin strips, w/fries:
  5 piece 77
  3 piece, 1 fish 100
  3 piece, shrimp 97
salads & lite catch:
  3 chicken, small salad 58
  1 fish, 2 chicken, small salad 96
  2 fish, small salad 119
  small salad 13
  shrimp and seafood salad 80
Create A Catch:
  chicken sandwich 82
  chicken strip 15
  fish sandwich 86
  fish sandwich, double 139
  fish fillet 53
  fries . . . . <2
  clam chowder cup 12
  clam chowder pint 24
  coleslaw, 5 oz. 50
sauces, 1 tbsp.:
  barbecue or cocktail 0

tartar sauce 4
salad dressing, 1 pkt.:
  blue cheese, premium 8
  Italian, gourmet or lo-cal 0
  ranch house 0
  Thousand Island 6

Sloppy joe seasoning:
  (Lawry's Seasoning Blends) 0
  mix *(French's)* 0
  mix *(McCormick/Schilling)* 0

Smelt, rainbow, meat only:
  raw, 1 lb. 318
  raw, 1 oz. 20
  baked, broiled, or microwaved, 4 oz. 102

Snack mix:
  (Eagle) 0
  (Flavor Tree Party Mix) 0
  (Ralston Chex Traditional) 0
  (Super Snax) 0
  plain or smoked *(Pepperidge Farm)* 0
  spicy *(Pepperidge Farm),* 1 oz. . . . . <5

Snail, sea, see "Whelk"

Snapper, meat only:
  raw, 1 lb. 168
  raw, 1 oz. 10
  baked, broiled, or microwaved, 4 oz. 53

Snow peas, see "Peas, edible-podded"

Soft drinks and mixers:
  nonmilk type, all flavors (all brands) 0

Sole:
  fresh, see "Flatfish"
  frozen *(Van de Kamp's* Natural), 4 oz. 35

Sole dinner, frozen:
  au gratin *(Healthy Choice)*, 11 oz. 55

Sole entrée, frozen:
  (Mrs. Paul's Light Fillets), 1 piece 50
  (Van de Kamp's Light), 1 piece 45
  in lemon butter *(Gorton's Microwave Entrees)*,
    1 pkg. 120
  w/lemon butter sauce *(Healthy Choice)*, 8.25 oz. . . 45
  in wine sauce *(Gorton's Microwave Entrees)*, 1 pkg. 90

Sorbet (see also "Sherbet" and "Ice"):
  all flavors *(Dole)* 0
  raspberry *(Frusen Glädjé)* 0

Sorghum:
  whole-grain 0

Sorghum syrup:
  1/2 cup 0

Sorrel, see "Dock"

Soup, canned, ready-to-serve, 9.5 oz., except as
  noted:
  bean:
    (Grandma Brown's), 1 cup . . . . <1
    w/ham *(Campbell's* Chunky Old Fashioned),
      9 5/8 oz. 0
    w/ham, chowder *(Hormel Micro-Cup* Hearty),
      1 pkg. 30
  beef, regular or hearty *(Progresso)* 35
  beef, w/mushrooms *(Campbell's* Chunky Low
    Sodium), 10.5 oz. 45
  beef barley *(Progresso)* 30
  beef broth, seasoned *(Progresso)*, 4 oz. 0
  beef minestrone *(Progresso)* 30
  beef noodle *(Progresso)* 40

The Cholesterol Content of Food

beef vegetable:
(Hormel Micro-Cup Hearty), 1 pkg. 9
(Lipton Hearty Ones), 1 pkg. 29
(Progresso) 35
borscht:
all varieties *(Gold's)* 0
all varieties *(Manischewitz)* 0
all varieties *(Rokeach)* 0
chickarina *(Progresso)* 20
chicken:
cream of *(Progresso)* 35
hearty *(Progresso)* 25
homestyle *(Progresso)* 20
chicken barley *(Progresso)*, 9.25 oz. 20
chicken broth:
(Campbell's Low Sodium), 10.5 oz. . . . . <5
(Hain/Hain No Salt), 8.75 oz. 5
(Progresso), 4 oz. . . . . <5
chicken minestrone *(Progresso)* 20
chicken mushroom, creamy *(Campbell's* Chunky),
9³/₈ oz. 50
chicken w/noodles *(Campbell's* Low Sodium),
10.5 oz. 65
chicken noodle:
(Hain) 20
(Hain No Salt) 25
(Hormel Micro-Cup Hearty), 1 pkg. 22
(Lipton Hearty Ones Homestyle), 11-oz. pkg. . . . 37
(Progresso) 40
chicken rice *(Campbell's* Chunky) 30
chicken rice *(Progresso)* 25
chicken vegetable:
(Campbell's Chunky) 25
(Progresso) 25
and rice *(Hormel Micro-Cup* Hearty), 1 pkg. . . . 7
clam chowder:
Manhattan *(Progresso)* 10
New England *(Hain)*, 9.25 oz. 25

213

Corinne T. Netzer

Soup, canned, ready-to-serve *(cont.)*

New England *(Hormel Micro-Cup* Hearty), 1 pkg.	30
corn chowder *(Progresso)*, 9.25 oz.	10
escarole in chicken broth *(Progresso)*, 9.25 oz.	<5
ham and bean *(Progresso)*	10
lentil:	
(Progresso)	0
w/sausage *(Progresso)*	20
vegetarian *(Hain/Hain* No Salt Added)	5
macaroni and bean *(Progresso)*	0
minestrone:	
(Campbell's Chunky)	0
(Hain/Hain No Salt Added)	0
(Health Valley), 7.5 oz.	0
(Hormel Micro-Cup Hearty), 1 pkg.	10
(Lipton Hearty Ones), 11-oz. pkg.	6
(Progresso)	0
hearty *(Progresso)*, 9.25 oz.	<5
zesty *(Progresso)*	10
mushroom:	
cream of *(Campbell's* Low Sodium), 10.5 oz.	20
cream of *(Progresso)*, 9.25 oz.	15
creamy *(Hain)*, 9.25 oz.	15
mushroom barley *(Hain)*	10
onion, French *(Campbell's* Low Sodium), 10.5 oz.	15
pea, split:	
(Grandma Brown's), 1 cup	<1
(Hain/Hain No Salt Added)	0
green *(Progresso)*	<5
w/ham *(Campbell's* Low Sodium), 10.5 oz.	10
w/ham *(Progresso)*	15
schav *(Gold's)*	15
tomato *(Progresso)*	0
tomato, w/tomato pieces *(Campbell's* Low Sodium), 10.5 oz.	10
tomato beef, w/rotini *(Progresso)*	30
tomato tortellini *(Progresso)*, 9.25 oz.	10
tortellini *(Progresso)*	10

tortellini, creamy *(Progresso)*, 9.25 oz.	35
turkey rice *(Hain)*	20
turkey rice *(Hain* No Salt Added)	15
vegetable:	
(Campbell's Chunky)	0
(Progresso)	<5
broth *(Hain/Hain* Low Sodium)	0
country *(Hormel Micro-Cup* Hearty), 1 pkg.	1
vegetarian *(Hain/Hain* No Salt Added)	0
vegetable beef:	
(Campbell's Chunky Low Sodium), 10.5 oz.	50
(Campbell's Chunky Old Fashioned)	25
vegetable chicken *(Hain)*	15
vegetable chicken *(Hain* No Salt Added)	20
vegetable pasta, Italian *(Hain/Hain* No Salt)	20

Soup, canned, condensed,[1] 8 oz., except as noted:

asparagus, cream of *(Campbell's)*	<5
bean w/bacon *(Campbell's)*	5
bean w/bacon *(Campbell's* Special Request)	5
beef:	
(Campbell's)	10
broth or bouillon *(Campbell's)*	0
consommé, w/gelatin *(Campbell's)*	0
beef noodle:	
(Campbell's)	15
(Campbell's Homestyle)	20
celery, cream of *(Campbell's)*	0
cheese, cheddar *(Campbell's)*	10
chicken, cream of *(Campbell's)*	10
chicken, cream of *(Campbell's* Special Request) . .	10
chicken alphabet *(Campbell's)*	10
chicken broth *(Campbell's)*	0
chicken broth and noodles *(Campbell's)*	10

[1] *Prepared according to package directions, with water, except as noted.*

Soup, canned, condensed *(cont.)*

chicken and dumplings *(Campbell's* Chicken 'n
  Dumplings 25
chicken gumbo *(Campbell's)* 5
chicken mushroom, creamy *(Campbell's)* 15
chicken noodle:
  (Campbell's/Campbell's Homestyle) 15
  (Campbell's Noodle-O's) 20
  (Campbell's Special Request) 15
chicken w/rice *(Campbell's)* 10
chicken w/rice *(Campbell's Special Request)* 10
chicken and stars *(Campbell's)* 10
chicken vegetable *(Campbell's)* 10
chili beef *(Campbell's)* 10
clam chowder:
  Manhattan *(Campbell's)* 0
  New England *(Campbell's)* 5
  New England, w/whole milk *(Campbell's)* 21
  New England, w/whole milk *(Gorton's)*, 1/4 can . . 15
minestrone *(Campbell's)* 0
mushroom:
  beefy *(Campbell's)* 10
  cream of *(Campbell's)* 0
  cream of *(Campbell's Special Request)* . . . . . . <5
  golden *(Campbell's)* . . . . <5
noodle, curly, w/chicken *(Campbell's)* 15
noodle and ground beef *(Campbell's)* 25
onion:
  cream of *(Campbell's)* 15
  cream of, w/water and whole milk *(Campbell's)* 23
  French *(Campbell's)* . . . . <5
oyster stew *(Campbell's)* 25
oyster stew, w/whole milk *(Campbell's)* 41
pea, green *(Campbell's)* 5
pea, split, w/ham and bacon *(Campbell's)* 5
pepper pot *(Campbell's)* 40
potato, cream of *(Campbell's)* 5

potato, cream of, w/water and whole milk
(Campbell's) 13
Scotch broth *(Campbell's)* 10
shrimp, cream of *(Campbell's)* 20
shrimp, cream of, w/whole milk *(Campbell's)* 36
tomato:
  (Campbell's/Campbell's Special Request) 0
  bisque *(Campbell's)* .... <5
  w/whole milk *(Campbell's)* 16
tomato, cream of *(Campbell's Homestyle)* ...... <5
tomato rice *(Campbell's Old Fashioned)* 0
turkey noodle *(Campbell's)* 15
turkey vegetable *(Campbell's)* 10
vegetable:
  (Campbell's) 0
  (Campbell's Homestyle/Old Fashioned) 0
  (Campbell's Special Request) .... <5
  Spanish style or vegetarian *(Campbell's)* 0
vegetable beef *(Campbell's)* 10
vegetable beef *(Campbell's Special Request)* 10
wonton *(Campbell's)* 10

Soup, frozen, 7.5 oz., except as noted:
all varieties, except broccoli, mushroom, spinach,
  or zucchini *(Tabatchnick)* 0
broccoli, cream of *(Tabatchnick)* 4
mushroom, cream of *(Tabatchnick)*, 6 oz. 3
spinach, cream of *(Tabatchnick)* 4
zucchini *(Tabatchnick)*, 6 oz. 3

Soup mix,[1] 6 fl. oz., except as noted:
broccoli, golden *(Lipton Cup-A-Soup Lite)* 1
chicken:
  broth *(Lipton Cup-A-Soup)* 1
  Florentine *(Lipton Cup-A-Soup Lite)* 6
  lemon *(Lipton Cup-A-Soup Lite)* 4

---

[1] *Prepared according to package directions, with water, except as noted.*

Soup mix, chicken *(cont.)*
   vegetable *(Lipton Cup-A-Soup)* 8
   onion *(Mrs. Grass* Soup & Dip Mix), 1/4 pkg. 0
   Oriental *(Lipton Cup-A-Soup Lite)* 3
   pea, split *(Manischewitz)* 0
   seafood chowder *(Golden Dipt)*, 1/4 pkg. dry 2
   shrimp bisque *(Golden Dipt)*, 1/4 pkg. dry 2
   tomato, creamy, and herb *(Lipton Cup-A-Soup
     Lite)* 2
   vegetable *(Manischewitz)* 0
   vegetable, spring *(Lipton Cup-A-Soup)* 6

Sour cream, see "Cream, sour"

Soursop:
   fresh 0

Soy flour:
   all varieties 0

Soy meal:
   all varieties 0

Soy milk:
   fluid or powder 0

Soy protein:
   all varieties 0

Soy sauce:
   (Kikkoman/Kikkoman Lite), 1 tbsp. . . . . tr.
   (La Choy/La Choy Lite) 0
   tamari or shoyu 0

Soybean:
   green or dried, plain 0

Soybean, fermented, see "Miso" and "Natto"

Soybean cake or curd, see "Tofu"

Soybean kernels:
all varieties   0

Spaghetti, see "Pasta"

Spaghetti dinner, frozen:
w/meat sauce *(Kid Cuisine),* 9.25 oz.   35
and meatballs *(Banquet),* 10 oz.   30
and meatballs *(Morton),* 10 oz.   10

Spaghetti dishes, mix*:
(Kraft American Style Dinner), 1 cup   0
Italian style, tangy *(Kraft* Dinner), 1 cup   5
w/meat sauce *(Kraft* Dinner), 1 cup   15

Spaghetti entrée, canned or packaged:
w/meatballs *(Chef Boyardee* Microwave), 7.5 oz. . . .   20
and meatballs, in sauce *(Buitoni),* 7.5 oz.   20

Spaghetti entrée, frozen:
w/beef *(Dining Lite),* 9 oz.   20
w/beef and mushroom sauce *(Lean Cuisine),*
11.5 oz.   25
w/beef sauce and mushrooms *(Le Menu*
LightStyle), 9 oz.   15
w/Italian sausage *(The Budget Gourmet),* 10 oz. . . .   48
w/meat sauce *(Healthy Choice),* 10 oz.   15
w/meat sauce *(Weight Watchers),* 10.5 oz.   25

Spaghetti sauce, see "Pasta sauce"

Spaghetti squash:
fresh, baked or boiled   0

Spaghettini entrée:
(Hormel Top Shelf), 1 serving   5

Spareribs, see "Pork"

Spinach:
fresh, canned, or frozen, plain 0
frozen:
creamed *(Birds Eye* Combinations), 3 oz. 0
creamed *(Green Giant)*, 1/2 cup 2
au gratin *(The Budget Gourmet)*, 6 oz. 40
in butter sauce *(Green Giant)*, 1/2 cup 5

Spinach, New Zealand, see "New Zealand spinach"

Spiny lobster, meat only:
raw, 1 lb. 318
raw, 1 oz. 20

Split peas:
boiled 0

Spring onion, see "Onion, green"

Sprouts, see "Bean sprouts"

Squab, meat only:
raw, breast, 1 oz. 26

Squash, all varieties:
fresh, canned, or frozen, w/out sauce 0

Squash seeds:
all varieties 0

Squid, meat only:
raw, 1 lb. 1059
raw, 1 oz. 66

Star fruit, see "Carambola"

The Cholesterol Content of Food

Steak sauce (see also specific listings):
(A.1.), 1 tbsp. 0
(French's), 1 tbsp. 0
(Heinz 57), 1 tbsp. 0
(Lea & Perrins), 1 oz. 0
(Steak Supreme), 1 tbsp. 0

Steak seasoning:
broiled *(McCormick/Schilling Spice Blends)* 0

Stir-fry sauce:
(Kikkoman) 0

Stomach, pork:
raw, 1 oz. 55

Strawberry:
fresh, canned, freeze-dried, or frozen 0

Strawberry drink or juice:
(all brands) 0

Strawberry flavor milk drink:
canned *(Sego/Sego Lite),* 10 oz. 5
mix *(Carnation Instant Breakfast),* 1 pkt. 3
mix *(Nestlé Quik),* 3/4 oz. or 2 1/2 heaping tsp. 0
mix *(Pillsbury Instant Breakfast),* 1 pkt. 0

Strawberry nectar:
(Libby's) 0

Strawberry topping:
(Kraft) 0
(Smucker's) 0

Strawberry yogurt dessert, frozen:
(Sara Lee Free & Light) 0

String beans, see "Green beans"

Stuffing, all varieties, 1 oz.:
  (Brownberry) 0
  (Pepperidge Farm/Pepperidge Farm Distinctive) . . 0

Stuffing mix:
  dry:
    (Croutettes), .7 oz. 0
    all varieties *(Golden Grain),* 1 oz. . . . . <1
    Cajun style *(Golden Dipt),* 1/4 cup 0
    cheddar and French *(Golden Dipt),* 1/4 cup 14
    garden herb *(Golden Dipt),* 1/4 cup 0
  prepared w/butter, 1/2 cup:
    all varieties *(Stove Top)* 20
    all varieties, except broccoli and cheese *(Stove
      Top* Microwave). 10
    all varieties *(Stove Top* Flexible Serving) 15
    broccoli and cheese *(Stove Top* Microwave) . . . 15
    San Francisco *(Stove Top Americana)* 20

Succotash:
  fresh, canned, or frozen, w/out sauce 0

Sucker, white, meat only:
  raw, 1 lb. 187
  raw, 1 oz. 12

Sugar, beet or cane:
  brown, granulated, or **confectioner's** 0

Sugar, maple:
  1-oz. piece 0

Sugar, substitute:
  all varieties (all brands) 0

Sugar apple:
  fresh 0

Sugar snap peas, see "Peas, edible-podded"

The Cholesterol Content of Food

Summer sausage (see also "Thuringer cervelat"):
  (Oscar Mayer), .8-oz. slice 19
  beef *(Oscar Mayer)*, .8-oz. slice 18

Sunfish, pumpkinseed, meat only:
  raw, 1 lb. 304
  raw, 1 oz. 19

Sunflower seed butter:
  all varieties 0

Sunflower seed flour:
  all varieties 0

Sunflower seeds:
  all varieties 0

Surimi (from Alaska walleye pollack):
  1 lb. 135
  1 oz. 9

Swamp cabbage:
  raw or boiled 0

Swedish sausage:
  (Hickory Farms), 1 oz. 20

Sweet potato:
  fresh, canned, or frozen, w/out sauce 0

Sweet potato leaf:
  raw or cooked 0

Sweet and sour cocktail mix:
  bottled *(Holland House)* 0

Sweet and sour sauce:
  (Kikkoman) 0
  (Sauceworks) 0

Sweet and sour sauce *(cont.)*
regular or duck sauce *(La Choy)* 0

Sweetbreads, see "Pancreas" and "Thymus"

Swiss chard:
fresh 0

Swiss steak, see "Beef dinner"

Swordfish, meat only:
fresh:
raw, 1 lb. 178
raw, 1 oz. 11
baked, broiled, or microwaved, 4 oz. 57
frozen, steaks w/out seasoning *(Sea-Pak),* 6 oz. . . 70

Syrup, see specific listings

Szechwan sauce:
hot and spicy *(La Choy)* 0

T

Food and Measure	Cholesterol (mgs.)
Tabbouleh mix:	
(Fantastic Foods)	0
(Near East)	0
salad (Casbah)	0
Taco Bell, 1 serving:	
burrito:	
bean, red sauce, 7.3 oz.	9
beef, red sauce, 7.3 oz.	57
chicken, no red sauce, 6 oz.	52
combination, 7 oz.	33
Supreme, 9 oz.	33
cinnamon twists, 1.2 oz.	0
Enchirito, red sauce, 7.5 oz.	54

Taco Bell *(cont.)*
Mexican pizza, 7.9 oz. 52
Meximelt, 3.7 oz. 38
Meximelt, chicken, 3.8 oz. 48
nachos:
  3.7 oz. 9
  BellGrande, 10.1 oz. 36
  Supreme, 5.1 oz. 18
pintos 'n cheese, red sauce, 4.5 oz. 16
taco:
  2.75 oz. 32
  BellGrande, 5.7 oz. 56
  chicken, 3 oz. 52
  chicken, soft, 3.8 oz. 52
  soft, 3.25 oz. 32
  steak, soft, 3.5 oz. 30
  Supreme, 3.25 oz. 32
  Supreme, soft, 4.4 oz. 32
taco salad, 21 oz. 80
taco salad, w/out shell, 18.3 oz. 80
tostada, red sauce, 5.5 oz. 16
tostada, chicken, red sauce, 5.8 oz. 37
sauces and condiments:
  green or red sauce 0
  guacamole 0
  nacho cheese, 2 oz. 9
  ranch dressing, 2.6 oz. 35
  salsa 0
  sour cream 0
  taco sauce, regular or hot 0

Taco dip:
(Wise) 0
and sauce *(Hain),* 4 tbsp. 5

Taco mix*:
vegetarian *(Natural Touch)* 0

Taco sauce:
all varieties *(Del Monte)* 0
all varieties *(La Victoria)* 0
all varieties *(Lawry's)* 0
all varieties *(Old El Paso)* 0
all varieties *(Ortega)* 0
mild *(Enrico's* No Salt Added) 0
mild or medium *(Heinz)* 0
red, mild *(El Molino)* 0

Taco seasoning mix:
(Hain) 0
(Lawry's Seasoning Blends) 0
(McCormick/Schilling) 0
(Old El Paso) 0
(Tio Sancho) 0
prepared w/meat *(Ortega)*, 1 oz. 20
salad *(Lawry's* Seasoning Blends) 0

Taco shell:
(Gebhardt) 0
(Ortega) 0
all sizes *(Lawry's)* 0
all sizes *(Old El Paso)* 0
all sizes *(Tio Sancho)* 0
corn *(Azteca)* 0

Tahini (see also "Sesame paste"):
from raw or roasted kernels 0
mix *(Casbah)* 0

Tamale, canned:
(Old El Paso), 2 pieces 20

Tamale dinner, frozen:
(Patio), 13 oz. 35

Tamarind:
fresh or dried 0

Tangerine:
fresh or canned 0

Tangerine juice:
fresh, canned, chilled, or frozen 0

Tapioca:
pearl, dry 0

Taro:
all varieties, raw or prepared, w/out sauce 0

Taro chips:
1/2 cup 0

Taro leaf or shoot:
raw or cooked 0

Tarragon:
fresh or dried (all brands) 0

Tart shell, see "Pastry shell"

Tartar sauce, 1 tbsp.:
(Golden Dipt) 10
(Golden Dipt Lite) 5
(Great Impressions) 10
(Hellmann's/Best Foods) 5
all varieties *(Sauceworks)* 5

Tea, brewed:
regular or instant, plain, flavored, or herbal (all
brands) 0

Tempeh:
all varieties 0

The Cholesterol Content of Food

Tempura batter mix:
  (Golden Dipt) 0

Teriyaki sauce:
  (Kikkoman), 1 tbsp. tr.
  (Kikkoman Baste & Glaze), 1 tbsp. 0
  (La Choy Thick & Rich), 1 oz. . . . . <1
  ginger marinade *(Golden Dipt)*, 1 fl. oz. 0

Thirst quencher drink:
  all flavors *(Gatorade)* 0

Thuringer cervelat (see also "Summer sausage"):
  beef and pork, 1 oz. 19

Thyme:
  fresh or dried (all brands) 0

Thymus:
  beef, braised, 4 oz. 333
  veal, braised, 4 oz. 532

Toaster muffins and pastries, 1 piece:
  apple-cinnamon *(Pepperidge Farm* Croissant
    Toaster Tarts) 0
  banana nut *(Thomas' Toast-r-Cakes)* 10
  cheese *(Pepperidge Farm* Croissant Toaster Tarts) 10
  oat bran, w/raisins *(Awrey's* Toastums) 0
  strawberry *(Pepperidge Farm* Croissant Toaster
    Tarts) 0

Tofu:
  raw, dried-frozen, grilled, okara, or fermented 0

Tofu dishes, see specific listings

Tofu patty, frozen:
  all varieties *(Natural Touch)* 0

Tofu spread, canned:
   all styles *(Natural Touch Tofu Topper)* 0

Tomatillo:
   (Frieda of California) 0

Tomato:
   fresh, canned, or pickled (all brands) 0

Tomato juice:
   (all brands) 0

Tomato paste:
   canned (all brands) 0

Tomato sauce, canned (see also "Pasta sauce,
   canned"):
   (S&W) 0
   (Stokely) 0
   all varieties *(Contadina)* 0
   all varieties *(Del Monte)* 0
   all varieties *(Hunt's)* 0
   all varieties *(Rokeach)* 0

Tomato sauce, refrigerated, see "Pasta sauce,
   refrigerated"

Tom Collins cocktail mix:
   bottled or instant *(Holland House)* 0

Tomato-chili cocktail:
   (Snap-E-Tom) 0

Tongue, fresh, braised:
   beef, 4 oz. 121
   lamb, 4 oz. 214
   pork, 4 oz. 166

The Cholesterol Content of Food

Tortellini, frozen or refrigerated:
egg or spinach, w/cheese *(Contadina Fresh)*,
  4.5 oz.   70
egg or spinach, w/chicken and prosciutto, or
  w/meat *(Contadina Fresh)*, 4.5 oz.   75
meatless or nondairy *(Tofutti)*   0

Tortellini dinner, frozen:
cheese *(Le Menu* LightStyle), 10 oz.   15

Tortellini entree, frozen:
cheese *(The Budget Gourmet* Side Dish), 5.5 oz. . . .   15
cheese *(Weight Watchers)*, 9 oz.   15
cheese, meat sauce and *(Le Menu* LightStyle),
  8 oz.   15
cheese, in tomato sauce *(Birds Eye For One)*,
  5.5 oz.   25
Provençale *(Green Giant* Microwave Garden
  Gourmet), 1 pkg.   15

Tortellini entree, packaged:
w/shrimp and seafood *(Hormel Top Shelf)*, 10 oz.   89
in marinara sauce *(Hormel Top Shelf)*, 10 oz.   35

Tortilla:
corn or flour, all sizes *(Azteca)*   0
corn or flour *(Old El Paso)*   0

Tortilla chips, see "Corn chips and similar snacks"

Tostaco shell:
(Old El Paso)   0

Tostada shell:
(Lawry's)   0
(Old El Paso)   0
(Ortega)   0
(Tio Sancho)   0

Tree fern:
raw or cooked 0

Triticale:
whole-grain or flour 0

Trout (see also "Sea trout"), meat only:
raw, 1 lb. 264
raw, 1 oz. 16
rainbow:
   raw, 1 lb. 257
   raw, 1 oz. 16
   baked, broiled, or microwaved, 4 oz. 83

Tuna, fresh, meat only:
bluefin:
   raw, 1 lb. 173
   raw, 1 oz. 11
   baked, broiled, or microwaved, 4 oz. 56
skipjack, raw, 1 lb. 213
skipjack, raw, 1 oz. 13
yellowfin, raw, 1 lb. 203
yellowfin, raw, 1 oz. 13

Tuna, canned, drained, 2 oz.:
solid light, in oil or water *(Star-Kist/Star-Kist* Prime
   Catch) 25
chunk light, in oil or water *(Bumble Bee)* 30
chunk light, in oil or water *(Star-Kist)* 25
solid white, albacore, in oil or water:
   (Bumble Bee) 30
   (Star-Kist) 25
chunk white, in oil or water *(Bumble Bee)* 30
chunk white, in oil or water *(Star-Kist)* 25

Tuna, frozen:
steak, w/out seasoning mix *(SeaPak),* 6 oz. 75

"Tuna," vegetarian, frozen:
(Worthington Tuno)   0

Tuna pie, frozen:
(Banquet), 7 oz.   30

Tuna salad:
(Longacre/Longacre Saladfest), 1 oz.   10

Turkey, fresh, all classes, roasted:
meat w/skin, 4 oz.   93
meat only, 4 oz.   86
meat only, diced, 1 cup   107
skin only, 1 oz.   32
light meat:
  w/skin, 4 oz.   86
  meat only, 4 oz.   78
  meat only, diced, 1 cup   97
dark meat:
  w/skin, 4 oz.   101
  meat only, 4 oz.   96
  meat only, diced, 1 cup   119
back, meat w/skin, 4 oz.   103
breast, meat w/skin:
  1/2 breast, 1.9 lb. (4.2 lbs. raw w/bone)   643
  4 oz.   84
leg, meat w/skin:
  1 leg, 1.2 lb. (1.5 lbs. raw w/bone)   466
  4 oz.   96
wing, meat w/skin:
  1 wing, 6.6 oz. (9.9 oz. raw w/bone)   150
  4 oz.   92

Turkey, canned, chunk:
white or white and dark *(Swanson),* 2 1/2 oz.   45

Turkey, frozen or refrigerated:
breast, raw *(Longacre* Cook-N-Bag), 1 oz.   10

Turkey, frozen or refrigerated *(cont.)*

breast, cooked:

(Land O'Lakes), 3 oz.	50
(Longacre Cook-N-Bag), 1 oz.	15
(Louis Rich), 1 oz.	21
barbecued or honey-roasted *(Louis Rich)*, 1 oz.	12
barbecue, quarter *(Mr. Turkey* Chub), 1 oz.	11
hen *(Louis Rich)*, 1 oz.	19
hickory smoked *(Louis Rich)*, 1 oz.	13
oven prepared, quarter *(Mr. Turkey Chub)*, 1 oz.	12
oven-roasted *(Louis Rich)*, 1 oz.	13
roast *(Louis Rich)*, 1 oz.	19
slices *(Louis Rich)*, 1 oz.	17
smoked *(Louis Rich)*, 1 oz.	11
smoked, quarter *(Mr. Turkey* Chub), 1 oz.	10
steaks *(Louis Rich)*, 1 oz.	17
tenderloins *(Louis Rich)*, 1 oz.	18
dark meat, skinless, roasted *(Swift Butterball)*, 3.5 oz.	130
drumstick or thigh *(Louis Rich)*, 1 oz. cooked	27
ground, see "Turkey, ground"	
white meat, skinless, roasted *(Swift Butterball)*, 3.5 oz.	80
white and dark meat w/skin, roasted *(Swift Butterball)*, 3.5 oz.	100
whole, cooked, w/out giblets *(Louis Rich)*, 1 oz.	22

wings:

(Louis Rich), 1 oz. cooked	31
(Louis Rich Drumettes), 1 oz. cooked	29
portions *(Louis Rich)*, 1 oz. cooked	29

young:

(Land O'Lakes), 3 oz.	65
butter basted *(Land O'Lakes)*, 3 oz.	85
self-basting, broth *(Land O'Lakes)*, 3 oz.	77

Turkey, ground (see also "Turkey kielbasa" and "Turkey sausage"):

(Longacre), 1 oz.	30

(Mr. Turkey), 1 oz.	20
cooked *(Louis Rich/Louis Rich* 90% Lean), 1 oz. . .	25
cooked, w/natural flavoring *(Louis Rich)*, 1 oz. . . .	24

Turkey, luncheon meat and boneless, cooked,
1 oz., except as noted:
bologna, see "Turkey bologna"
breast:

(Healthy Deli Gourmet/Lessalt)	9
(Longacre Salt Watchers)	15
(Mr. Turkey)	10
all styles *(Longacre Premium)*	10
all styles *(Longacre Deli Chef)*	15
honey *(Healthy Deli)*	9
honey-roasted or oven-roasted *(Louis Rich)*. . . .	11
golden *(Boar's Head)*	20
golden, skinless *(Boar's Head)*	10
oven-cooked *(Healthy Deli)*	8
oven-roasted *(Eckrich Lite)*	10
oven-roasted *(Louis Rich* Thin Sliced), .4-oz. slice	4
oven-roasted *(Oscar Mayer)*, .7-oz. slice	9
roast *(Louis Rich)*	20
roast *(Oscar Mayer* Thin Sliced), .4-oz. slice . . .	5

breast, smoked:

(Eckrich Lite)	10
(Healthy Deli)	8
(Healthy Deli Gourmet)	11
(Longacre)	15
(Louis Rich), .7-oz. slice	9
(Louis Rich Thin Sliced), .4-oz. slice	5
(Mr. Turkey)	10
(Oscar Mayer), .7-oz. slice	9
sliced *(Longacre)*	10
breast and white *(Longacre Deli Chef)*	15

ham, see "Turkey ham"

luncheon loaf *(Louis Rich)*	16
luncheon loaf, spiced *(Mr. Turkey)*	11

Turkey, luncheon meat and boneless *(cont.)*
  pastrami, see "Turkey pastrami"
  salami, see "Turkey salami"
  sausage, see "Turkey sausage"
  smoked *(Louis Rich)* 14

"Turkey," vegetarian:
  canned or frozen, all varieties *(Worthington)* 0

Turkey bacon, see "Bacon, substitute"

Turkey bologna:
  (Longacre Sliced), 1 oz. 25
  (Louis Rich), 1 oz. 22
  mild *(Louis Rich)*, 1 oz. 18

Turkey and corned beef:
  (Healthy Deli Doubledecker), 1 oz. 12

Turkey dinner, frozen:
  (Banquet), 10.5 oz. 40
  (Banquet Extra Helping), 19 oz. 65
  (Morton), 10 oz. 45
  breast:
    (Healthy Choice), 10.5 oz. 45
    Dijon *(The Budget Gourmet)*, 11.2 oz. 65
    sliced *(The Budget Gourmet)*, 11.1 oz. 45
    sliced, in mushroom sauce *(Lean Cuisine)*, 8 oz. 50
  divan *(Le Menu* LightStyle), 10 oz. 60
  w/dressing and gravy *(Armour Classics)*, 11.5 oz. 50
  sliced *(Le Menu* LightStyle), 10 oz. 30

Turkey entrée, frozen:
  à la king, w/rice *(The Budget Gourmet)* 10 oz. . . . 75
  breast, stuffed *(Weight Watchers)*, 8.5 oz. 80
  Dijon *(Lean Cuisine)*, 9.5 oz. 60
  glazed *(The Budget Gourmet* Slim Selects), 9 oz. 50
  glazed *(Le Menu* LightStyle), 8.25 oz. 35

pie:
  (Banquet), 7 oz. 40
  (Banquet Supreme Microwave), 7 oz. 35
  (Morton), 7 oz. 40
  sliced, breast, in mushroom sauce *(Lean Cuisine)*,
    8 oz. 50
  sliced, in curry sauce, w/rice pilaf *(Right Course)*,
    8.75 oz. 50
  traditional *(Le Menu* LightStyle), 8 oz. 25

Turkey fat:
  1 tbsp. 13

Turkey frankfurter:
  (Longacre), 1 oz. 30
  (Louis Rich), 1.6 oz. 42
  (Louis Rich Bun Length), 2 oz. 53
  (Mr. Turkey), 1.6 oz. 31
  cheese *(Louis Rich)*, 1.6 oz. 44
  cheese *(Mr. Turkey)*, 1.6 oz. 29

Turkey giblets, simmered:
  4 oz. 474
  chopped or diced, 1 cup 606

Turkey ham, 1 oz., except as noted:
  (Longacre Deli Lean Lite) 25
  *(Louis Rich-*round or unsliced) 19
  *(Louis Rich-*square), .7-oz. slice 14
  (Louis Rich Thin Sliced), .4-oz. slice 7
  breakfast, smoked *(Mr. Turkey)* 16
  buffet style or chopped *(Mr. Turkey)* 17
  chopped *(Louis Rich)* 19
  chunk *(Longacre)* 25
  honey cured *(Louis Rich)*, .7 oz. 14
  sliced *(Longacre)* 20
  smoked *(Mr. Turkey)* 18
  smoked *(Mr. Turkey* Chub) 17

Turkey and ham:
  (Healthy Deli Doubledecker), 1 oz.   11

Turkey ham salad:
  (Longacre/Longacre Saladfest), 1 oz.   10

Turkey kielbasa (see also "Turkey sausage"):
  (Louis Rich Polska), 1 oz.   19

Turkey nuggets:
  breaded *(Louis Rich),* .7-oz. heated piece   9

Turkey pastrami:
  (Louis Rich-round), 1 oz.   18
  (Louis Rich-square), .8-oz. slice   14
  (Louis Rich Thin Sliced), .4-oz. slice   7
  (Mr. Turkey), 1 oz.   17
  sliced *(Longacre),* 1 oz.   20

Turkey patty:
  breaded *(Louis Rich),* 2.8-oz. heated patty   32

Turkey pie, see "Turkey entree"

Turkey salad, 1 oz.:
  (Longacre)   10
  (Longacre Saladfest)   15

Turkey salami:
  (Longacre Sliced), 1 oz.   20
  (Louis Rich), 1 oz.   20
  cooked, 1 oz.   23
  cotto *(Louis Rich),* 1 oz.   21
  cotto *(Mr. Turkey),* 1 oz.   16

Turkey sausage (see also "Turkey kielbasa"):
  breakfast *(Mr. Turkey),* 1 oz.   16
  breakfast, ground, cooked *(Louis Rich),* 1 oz.   22
  breakfast links, cooked *(Louis Rich),* 1 link   18

Polish *(Louis Rich* Polska), 1 oz.   20
Polish *(Mr. Turkey* Polska), 1 oz.   15
smoked:
   (Louis Rich), 1 oz.   19
   (Mr. Turkey), 1 oz.   19
   w/cheese *(Louis Rich)*, 1 oz.   18

Turkey spread:
chunky *(Underwood* Light), 2$\frac{1}{8}$ oz.   25

Turkey sticks:
breaded *(Louis Rich)*, 1-oz. heated stick   12

Turkey summer sausage:
(Louis Rich), 1 oz.   21

Turmeric, ground:
(all brands)   0

Turnip:
fresh, canned, or frozen, w/out sauce   0

Turnip greens:
fresh, canned, or frozen, w/out sauce   0

Turnover, refrigerated:
apple or cherry *(Pillsbury)*   0

V

Food and Measure	Cholesterol (mgs.)
Vanilla extract:	
(Virginia Dare)	0
Vanilla flavor drink:	
canned, all varieties (Sego/Sego Lite), 10 oz.	5
Veal, meat only, 4 oz.:	
cubed, lean only, braised or stewed	164
ground, broiled	117
leg:	
braised, lean w/fat	152
braised, lean only	159
fried, lean w/fat	119
fried, lean only	121

roasted, lean w/fat	117
roasted, lean only	117
loin:	
braised, lean w/fat	134
braised, lean only	142
roasted, lean w/fat	117
roasted, lean only	120
rib:	
braised, lean w/fat	158
braised, lean only	163
roasted, lean w/fat	125
roasted, lean only	130
shoulder, whole:	
braised, lean w/fat	143
braised, lean only	147
roasted, lean w/fat	128
roasted, lean only	129
shoulder, arm:	
braised, lean w/fat	168
braised, lean only	176
roasted, lean w/fat	122
roasted, lean only	124
shoulder, blade:	
braised, lean w/fat	174
braised, lean only	179
roasted, lean w/fat	133
roasted, lean only	135
sirloin:	
braised, lean w/fat	122
braised, lean only	128
roasted, lean w/fat	116
roasted, lean only	118

Veal dinner, frozen:

marsala *(Le Menu* LightStyle), 10 oz.	75
parmigiana *(Armour Classics),* 11.25 oz.	55
parmigiana *(Morton),* 10 oz.	35

Corinne T. Netzer

Veal entrée, frozen:
  parmigiana, patty *(Weight Watchers)*, 8.44 oz. 55
  primavera *(Lean Cuisine)*, 9 1/8 oz. 80

Vegetable entrée:
  canned, chow mein, meatless *(La Choy)*, 3/4 cup . . 0
  frozen, and pasta Mornay, w/ham *(Lean Cuisine)*,
    9 3/8 oz. 35

Vegetable juice:
  all blends (all brands) 0

Vegetable sticks, frozen:
  (Stilwell Quickkrisp), 3 oz. . . . . <1

Vegetables, see specific listings

Vegetables, mixed:
  all varieties, canned or frozen, w/out sauce (all
    brands) 0
  frozen, prepared w/out added ingredients:
    in butter sauce *(Stokely Singles)*, 3 oz. 0
    in butter sauce *(Green Giant)*, 1/2 cup 5
    w/herb sauce for chicken or shrimp *(Birds Eye
      Custom Cuisine)*, 4.6 oz. 0
    w/mushroom sauce for beef *(Birds Eye Custom
      Cuisine)*, 4.6 oz. 5
    w/mustard sauce, Dijon, for chicken or fish *(Birds
      Eye Custom Cuisine)*, 4.6 oz. 5
    w/onion sauce *(Birds Eye Combinations)*, 2.6 oz. 0
    w/Oriental sauce for beef *(Birds Eye Custom
      Cuisine)*, 4.6 oz. 0
    pasta primavera style *(Birds Eye International)*,
      3.3 oz. 5
    w/rice in teriyaki sauce *(Stokely Singles)*, 4 oz. . . 0
    w/rotini in cheddar sauce *(Stokely Singles)*, 4 oz. 10
    w/shells in Italian style sauce *(Stokely Singles)*,
      4 oz. 5

242

w/tomato basil sauce for chicken *(Birds Eye
  Custom Cuisine)*, 4.6 oz. 0
w/white and wild rice pilaf *(Stokely Singles)*, 4 oz. 5
w/wild rice in wine sauce for chicken *(Birds Eye
  Custom Cuisine)*, 4.6 oz. 0

Vegetarian entrée, frozen (see also specific listings):
  (Natural Touch Dinner Entree) 0

Vegetarian foods, see specific listings

Venison, meat only:
  roasted, 4 oz. 127

Vienna sausage, canned:
  beef and pork, 2″ link, .6 oz. 8

Vine spinach:
  fresh 0

Vinegar:
  all varieties (all brands) 0

W

Food and Measure	Cholesterol (mgs.)
Waffle, frozen, 1 piece:	
(Aunt Jemima Original)	6
(Eggo Homestyle)	10
(Eggo Nutri · Grain)	0
(Roman Meal)	2
all varieties, except Hot-N-Buttery *(Downyflake)*	0
apple cinnamon *(Aunt Jemima)*	6
blueberry *(Aunt Jemima)*	5
buttermilk *(Aunt Jemima)*	7
buttermilk *(Eggo)*	10
oat bran, all varieties *(Eggo Common Sense)*	0
oat bran or whole-grain wheat *(Aunt Jemima)*	0
raisin and bran *(Eggo Nutri · Grain)*	0

Waffle, mix, see "Pancake and waffle mix"

Waffle breakfast, frozen:
Belgian *(Weight Watchers),* 1.5 oz.   5

Walnut:
black, English, or Persian   0

Walnut topping:
in syrup *(Smucker's)*   0

Water chestnut, Chinese:
fresh or canned   0

Watercress:
fresh   0

Watermelon:
fresh   0

Watermelon seeds:
dried, kernels   0

Wax beans:
fresh, canned, or frozen, plain (all brands)   0

Wax gourd:
raw or cooked   0

Wendy's, 1 serving:
Big Classic, 9.2 oz.   80
cheeseburger:
  bacon, Jr., 5.5 oz.   50
  Jr., 4.4 oz.   35
  Kids' Meal, 4.1 oz.   35
  Swiss Deluxe, Jr., 5.8 oz.   40
chicken:
  breast fillet, 3.5 oz.   65

Wendy's, chicken *(cont.)*

club sandwich, 7.2 oz.	70
fillet, grilled, 2.5 oz.	55
nuggets, crispy, 6 pieces	50
sandwich, grilled, 6.2 oz.	60
chicken nuggets sauces, all varieties	0
chili, regular, 9 oz.	45
fish fillet sandwich, 6 oz.	50
french fries, small, 3.2 oz.	0
hamburger:	
Jr., 3.9 oz.	35
Kids' Meal, 3.7 oz.	35
1/4 lb.	65
single, plain, 4.4 oz.	65
single, w/everything, 7.4 oz.	70
potato, baked, hot stuffed:	
plain, 8.8 oz.	0
bacon and cheese, 12.8 oz.	20
broccoli and cheese, 12.3 oz.	tr.
cheese, 11.2 oz.	10
chili and cheese, 14.2 oz.	25
sour cream and chives, 11.4 oz.	25
steak sandwich, country fried, 5.1 oz.	35
salads:	
chef, 9.1 oz.	40
garden, 8.1 oz.	0
taco, 17.3 oz.	35
salad dressings and condiments, 1 tbsp.:	
bacon-tomato dressing, reduced calorie	<1
blue cheese dressing	10
celery seed dressing	5
French dressing, regular or sweet red	0
Hidden Valley Ranch dressing	5
honey mustard	5
Italian dressing, golden or reduced calorie	0
Italian Caesar dressing	5
Thousand Island dressing	5

The Cholesterol Content of Food

salad bar, *Garden Spot:*

bacon bits, .5 oz.	10
breadsticks, .3 oz.	0
cheddar chips, 1 oz.	5
cheese, shredded (imitation), 1 oz.	tr.
chicken salad, 2 oz.	tr.
chow mein noodles, .5 oz.	0
coleslaw, 2 oz.	5
cottage cheese, 3.7 oz.	15
egg, hard cooked, .7 oz.	90
fruit, plain, all varieties	0
garbanzo beans (chick-peas), 1 oz.	0
Parmesan cheese, grated, 1 oz.	20
Parmesan cheese (imitation), grated, 1 oz.	tr.
pasta salad, 2 oz.	0
pepperoni, sliced, 1 oz.	35
potato salad, 2 oz.	10
pudding, butterscotch or chocolate, 2 oz.	tr.
seafood salad, 2 oz.	tr.
sunflower seeds and raisins, 1 oz.	0
tuna salad, 2 oz.	tr.
turkey ham, 1 oz.	15
vegetables, plain, all varieties	0

Superbar, Mexican:

cheese sauce, 2 oz.	tr.
refried beans, 2 oz.	tr.
rice, Spanish, 2 oz.	tr.
sour topping (imitation), 1 oz.	0
taco chips, 1.4 oz.	0
taco meat, 2 oz.	25
taco sauce, 1 oz.	tr.
taco shell, .4 oz.	0

Superbar, pasta:

Alfredo sauce, 2 oz.	tr.
fettuccine, 2 oz.	10
garlic toast, .6 oz.	tr.
pasta medley, 2 oz.	tr.
ravioli, cheese, in spaghetti sauce, 2 oz.	5

Wendy's, Superbar, pasta *(cont.)*
rotini, 2 oz.	tr.
spaghetti sauce, 2 oz.	tr.
spaghetti sauce, w/meat, 2 oz.	10
tortellini, cheese, in spaghetti sauce, 2 oz.	5

Western dinner, frozen:
(Banquet), 11 oz.	90
(Morton), 10 oz.	35

Wheat:
all varieties	0

Wheat, parboiled, see "Bulgur"

Wheat bran:
crude or processed (all brands)	0

Wheat cake:
(Quaker Grain Cakes)	0

Wheat flour:
all varieties (all brands)	0

Wheat germ:
all varieties *(Kretschmer)*	0

Wheat gluten:
vital *(Arrowhead Mills)*	0

Wheat pilaf mix:
(Casbah)	0

Whelk, meat only, raw:
1 lb.	294
1 oz.	18

Whey:
sweet, dry, 1 oz.	2
sweet, fluid, 1 cup	5

The Cholesterol Content of Food

Whiskey, see "Liquor"

Whiskey sour cocktail mix:
bottled or instant *(Holland House)*   0

White bean:
boiled, dried, or canned, w/out sauce   0

White sauce mix:
1³/4-oz. pkt. . . . .   tr.

Whitefish, meat only:
raw, 1 lb.   272
raw, 1 oz.   17
smoked, 4 oz.   37

Whiting, meat only:
raw, 1 lb.   303
raw, 1 oz.   19
baked, broiled, or microwaved, 4 oz.   95

Wild rice:
raw or cooked, w/out butter or sauce   0

Wild rice dishes, see "Rice dishes"

Wine:
all varieties (all brands)   0

Wine, cooking:
all varieties (all brands)   0

Winged bean:
fresh or dried   0

Wolf fish, Atlantic, meat only:
raw, 1 lb.   209
raw, 1 oz.   13

Wonton skin:
  (Nasoya)   0

Worcestershire sauce:
  all varieties *(Lea & Perrins)*   0
  regular or smoky *(French's)*   0

Y

Food and Measure	Cholesterol (mgs.)
Yam:	
all varieties, fresh, canned or frozen, w/out sauce	0
Yam bean tuber:	
raw or cooked	0
Yardlong bean:	
fresh or dried	0
Yeast, baker's:	
(all brands)	0
Yellow beans:	
dried	0

Yellow squash, see "Crookneck squash"

Yogurt, 8 oz., except as noted:
  plain:
    (Bison Lowfat), 1 cup 10
    (Bison Nonfat), 1 cup 0
    (Breyers Lowfat) 20
    (Colombo Nonfat Lite) 5
    (Crowley), 1 cup 30
    (Crowley Lowfat), 1 cup 10
    (Crowley Nonfat), 1 cup . . . . <1
    (Dannon Lowfat) 15
    (Dannon Nonfat) 5
    (Friendship Lowfat), 1 cup 14
    (Knudsen) 35
    (Knudsen Lowfat) 25
    (Yoplait), 6 oz. 15
  all flavors:
    (Colombo Nonfat Lite) 5
    (Dannon Fresh Flavors) 10
    (Light N'Lively Free), 4.4 oz. 0
    except blueberry, cherry, raspberry, or
      strawberry *(Knudsen Cal 70),* 6 oz. 0
    except lemon, peach, or strawberry *(Light*
      N'Lively 100) 0
  all fruit flavors:
    (Breyers Lowfat) 10
    (Crowley Nonfat), 1 cup . . . . <1
    (Crowley Sundae Style), 1 cup 10
    (Crowley Swiss Style), 1 cup 10
    (Dannon Extra Smooth), 4.4 oz. 10
    (Dannon Fruit-on-the-Bottom) 10
    (Dannon Hearty Nuts & Raisins) 10
    (Knudsen Lowfat) 15
    (Ripple 70), 6 oz. 5
    (Yoplait), 6 oz. 10
    (Yoplait Fat Free), 6 oz. 5
    (Yoplait Light), 6 oz. . . . . <5

(Yoplait Breakfast Yogurt), 6 oz.	20
(Yoplait Custard Style), 6 oz.	20
blueberry *(Light N' Lively)*	10
blueberry, cherry, raspberry, or strawberry *(Knudsen Cal 70)*, 6 oz.	5
cherry, black *(Light N' Lively)*	15
coffee or lemon *(Bison Lowfat)*, 1 cup	10
coffee *(Friendship Lowfat)*, 1 cup	14
lemon, peach, or strawberry *(Light N' Lively 100)*	5
peach *(Light N' Lively)*	15
pineapple or red raspberry *(Light N' Lively)*	10
piña colada *(Yoplait)*, 6 oz.	10
strawberry or strawberry fruit cup *(Light N' Lively)*	15
strawberry-banana *(Light N' Lively)*	10
vanilla:	
(Bison Lowfat), 1 cup	10
(Breyers Lowfat)	20
(Crowley Lowfat), 1 cup	10
(Dannon Hearty Nuts & Raisins)	10
(Friendship Lowfat), 1 cup	14
(Knudsen Lowfat)	15
(Yoplait), 6 oz.	15
(Yoplait Custard Style), 6 oz.	20
(Yoplait Fat Free), 6 oz.	<5
Yogurt, frozen, 3 fl. oz., except as noted:	
all flavors *(Dreyer's Inspirations)*, 3 oz.	5
all flavors *(Sealtest Free)*, 1/2 cup	0
all flavors, except vanilla *(Breyers)*, 1/2 cup	10
caramel pecan chunk *(Colombo Gourmet)*	10
cheesecake, wild raspberry *(Colombo Gourmet)*	5
cherry *(Crowley)*	5
chocolate:	
(Bison), 3.5 fl. oz.	5
(Crowley)	10
(Häagen-Dazs)	25
chunk, Bavarian *(Colombo Gourmet)*	10
Heath bar crunch *(Colombo Gourmet)*	15

Yogurt, frozen *(cont.)*

mocha Swiss almond *(Colombo* Gourmet)	10
peach *(Crowley)*	5
peach *(Häagen-Dazs)*	31
peanut butter cup *(Colombo* Gourmet)	5
raspberry *(Crowley)*	5
strawberry:	
(Crowley)	5
(Häagen-Dazs)	29
passion *(Colombo* Gourmet)	5
vanilla:	
(Breyers), 1/2 cup	15
(Crowley)	10
(Häagen-Dazs)	36
dream *(Colombo* Gourmet)	10
vanilla almond crunch *(Häagen-Dazs)*	33

Yogurt, frozen, soft-serve, all flavors:

(Bresler's Gourmet), 1 oz.	2
(Bresler's Lite), 1 oz.	0
(Crowley Peaks of Perfection), 3.5 fl. oz.	5
(Dannon), 4 fl. oz.	5
(Dannon Nonfat), 4 fl. oz.	0

Yogurt drink:

all flavors *(Dan'up)*, 8 oz.	10

Z

Food and Measure	Cholesterol (mgs.)
Ziti, frozen:	
in marinara sauce *(The Budget Gourmet* Side Dish), 6.25 oz.	15
Zucchini:	
fresh, canned, or frozen, w/out sauce	0
canned, w/tomato juice *(Del Monte),* 1/2 cup	0
canned, Italian style *(Progresso),* 1/2 cup	<1
frozen, breaded *(Stilwell Quickkrisp),* 3.3 oz.	15
frozen, w/carrots, pearl onions, and mushrooms *(Birds Eye* Farm Fresh), 4 oz.	0